Your Secret Weapon

The New Ultimate Marketing Plan
For Cosmetic Plastic Surgeons

VICTOR URBINA

Published by Urbina Media Group
3001 E Paisano Dr, El Paso, TX 79905, U.S.A.

Your Secret Weapon - The New Ultimate Marketing Plan For Cosmetic Plastic Surgeons - 1st ed.

ISBN-10: 0692556818
ISBN-13: 978-0692556818
LCCN: 2015917371

Printed in the United States of America

DEDICATION

I dedicate this book to my wife Georgialina and my parents Amado & Rosa Urbina. You have all been instrumental in the success I've enjoyed throughout my life. I thank each one of you for accepting my flaws and loving me for the man I have become.

Los quiero con todo mi corazón y agradezco a dios por tenerlos en mi vida. Ustedes hacen todo esto posible.

CONTENTS

Acknowledgments   i

Foreword   iii

Introduction   v

A Different Perspective   1

Why Current Marketing Efforts Aren't Enough   15

It's A System   27

A Few Tips And Tricks   33

How To Sell Without Selling   47

A Cultural Transformation   57

How To Find The Right Marketing Partner   63

Book Recap, i.e. 'Cliff Notes'   77

Final Thoughts   91

About the Author   95

ACKNOWLEDGMENTS

I would like to thank Dr. Guy Danielson for his contributions to this book, words of advice, and guidance throughout. My managers and employees at my "brick and mortar" retail stores for keeping the ship on course and allowing me to entertain and then actively pursue this new venture. My countless mentors, friends, relatives, and associates for always having a kind word of encouragement.

Baba Booey!

Foreword

Why is this book valuable and what are the skills that the author has acquired to make you successful in the cosmetic surgery arena? This is a book about forward thinking and execution. Written by a man that has mastered the most difficult and challenging aspect of excelling in a progressively more competitive world. It is centered on the principles of direct marketing; the only kind of marketing that could possibly help differentiate your practice. The genius of direct marketing is that it targets only the exact potential patients that you want to reach and serve. It is a process that employs feedback loops to constantly refine and improve your relationship with your ideal patient and in doing so attract more of them.

In preparing this message I've read Victor's book in successive drafts and have also read some of the numerous books on this topic and spent many hours evaluating the marketing tactics that are presently being used. What I discovered can be best summarized by saying, "The more I read and experience about the marketing of cosmetic surgery the less I am able to intelligently choose a surgeon." It is literally a sea of doctors with virtually no information that would allow any of the hundreds of surgeons in an area to stand out. To be blunt, all these doctors relying on "branding" and touting their superiority are missing the boat.

I am a neurosurgeon who has been in the practice of neurosurgery for over 40 years in the same location. In 2002 a vision formulated process I began in the mid 1990's culminated in a 40-bed multi disciplinary specialty hospital opening. Today that hospital is one of the top 10 in the US and at the top of the hospitals list in Texas. I am the author of a number one bestselling book and am constantly anticipating trends and never satisfied with the status quo. My approach for everything I have ever done is one of constant forward planning and changing. My guiding strategy is, "obsolete yourself before some else does it for you." Why do I mention any of these things? It's not to build myself up before you, or to brag, it's to let you know that I understand the amount of work that goes into being successful and therefore feel qualified to speak on the topic.

Those of us that undertake the journey to constantly enhance our own creative abilities, in order to prosper and succeed, are going to need to team up with other equally devoted, driven, and evolving experts in collaborative and synergetic ways to get to, and remain, at the top of our field. Only this will allow continuous growth and the ability to create equity in an organization that can evolve into a business that has value beyond the surgeons' own limited ability. In other words to progress from "employee with a job" to "owner" of a valuable asset that is independent of ones own necessity to be the producer. It's all about the desire for achievement and the mind set of each of us to decide if we are willing to make this commitment to ourselves.

Victor is one of us, who is on a similar path and the skills that he has mastered are mutually advantageous to your endeavors. What makes someone excel at being successful as a surgeon or a marketing guru are precisely the same. You must believe in yourself. Pick your goals. And treat all you contact with kindness, dignity, and respect. Furthermore, you can never give up your relentless commitment to achieve despite all odds, fears, and failures that will be inevitably encountered along the journey.

The bottom line is this. If you don't see yourself as an entrepreneur then this book isn't for you. If on the other hand you see yourself that way then Victor is a worthy and like-minded individual. And this book is evidence of his willingness to team up with you and become a prized asset on your journey.

- Guy Danielson, MD

Introduction

"Business has only two functions – marketing and innovation.
All the rest are costs."
– Peter Drucker

A buyer is a buyer is a buyer is a buyer. We all buy things for the same reasons—to fill some deep down emotional void that we have and need desperately to fill. There is a belief among many people—me included—that nature hates a void and will fill it almost immediately with something.

Think about it for a second how quickly have you filled a void in your life almost without even realizing it?

Ask any business owner what their number one business challenge is and nine out of 10 will give you the same answer: They want more leads and more customers. This tune is not new and it's one that will definitely not change anytime soon.

From the beginning of time, merchants tried a variety of different things to attract customers to their goods, and thus marketing was born. It is the most important activity in any business, because nothing happens until a customer walks in the door. Up until that point all you have is a very expensive hobby.

I struggled with new customer attraction for years in my business, and at times I'm still stumped, when it comes to getting people in the door.

Today, I am a UPS Store franchisee. I own stores throughout the country and have spent the better part of my life in or around some sort of entrepreneurial venture.

It all started when I was eight or nine years old and my father took me to his business, a watch store, and paid me per piece to set the time on bulk orders of watches. It continued into junior high when I would spend summers selling sodas out of an ice chest during the hot summers on south El Paso Street in El Paso, Texas.

I worked my way through high school and college, became a mechanical engineer, and earned a master's in business administration. I've worked for some of the biggest companies in the world. But throughout it all, I still felt unfulfilled.

After a few years, I left a very good, secure, high-paying job and came back to El Paso to begin my entrepreneurial journey. I was searching for a business idea and by sheer luck I stumbled across UPS Store franchises and became a franchisee. That decision has completely changed my life, for the better.

This book is for business owners—and, yes, you are a business owner—who are struggling to find a way to achieve autonomy and break the work-money link. Just because you're a physician and took the Hippocratic Oath doesn't mean you're not a business owner. If you hire and fire people, if people depend on you for a paycheck, if you worry about competition, then guess what? You're a business owner.

This book is for you if you are:
- Progressive and forward thinking.
- Viewed as a leader in your field.
- Not afraid to take calculated risk in order to get ahead.
- Not afraid to learn new things.
- Tired of working long hours for only slightly more or even flat practice growth.

My goal is to help you, the cosmetic practice owner, leapfrog years of painful and expensive trial and error.

I encourage you to learn from my mistakes. In the nine years that I have been in business, I estimate that I have spent upwards of $200,000 on marketing that just didn't work. I want to act as your guide to help you navigate the minefield of marketing as if you were wearing X-ray glasses. After reading this book you should have at least one immediately actionable and implementable marketing tactic for your practice. It might be a lost customer reactivation strategy, a referral strategy, or a lead generation strategy.

I am even willing to give you a written double your money back guarantee plus $100 if you read through the entire book and don't find a single idea worthwhile. I give you such a strong guarantee on the content of this book because I am that confident about what I have to tell you.

WHY AM I QUALIFIED TO GIVE SURGEONS ADVICE?

What does a UPS Store owner have in common with a cosmetic surgeon? Well, believe it or not, there are a lot of similarities between us. Let me explain.

If you choose to believe that your business is different because you're a physician and I'm a retailer, then read no further. If, however, you're open to getting a fresh, new take on your business, keep reading.

For the first few years I was in business, I was crushing it; business was more than I could handle at times, and life was good. I thought I was the Steve Jobs of retail.

So what does one do when they think they have it all figured out? They expand. And expand I did, but maybe a little too much. What I didn't realize was that the reason my first business was so successful was that I had a phenomenal location. I had no competition and, thus, had no need to advertise; the market was all mine.

After I expanded, I realized that I wasn't the only game in town and that I had to start marketing my business. If you're as successful early in your career as I was, chances are, you don't take the time to learn or sharpen your skills. Instead, I started "marketing" my stores—I use that word liberally because, looking back, all I was really doing was throwing away tons of cash.

Then one January day, I realized I had about six months of money left in the bank before I would be out of business. It was the wake-up call all business owners hate getting. I had to completely change the way I did business. I had to learn how to effectively and profitably market my stores.

After one year of intense study, frenetic implementation, and countless sleepless nights, I was able to put my stores in a secure financial position. Today, we have had continued growth for two straight years.

I still made my fair share of marketing mistakes, which were a welcome outcome because they allowed me to correct my course, but I've had far more verifiable wins than losses in all of my marketing efforts.

In this book, I'm going to share both my wins and my losses so that you can see that I'm not a consultant, but like you, I'm a real business owner with a real payroll to meet every other Friday.

I wrote this book because I see a huge gap in the marketing landscape for cosmetic practices. It seems that everyone is touting search engine optimization (SEO), Facebook, email marketing, and branding. Amazon lists at least a half dozen different books directed at online marketing for aesthetic plastic surgeons. Don't get me wrong, I think that these are key components of an effective marketing strategy, but to rely solely upon them is a huge mistake. For example, Facebook recently changed its ad policies to shut down many successful marketing campaigns, and Google is constantly changing its algorithms, making SEO reliant on the whims of techno geeks comfortably employed and not fighting for a dollar the way you and I are.

There is a breadth of opportunity with a medium that is getting less crowded every day. I'm talking about offline marketing. That's right, the tried-and-true reliable world of direct mail and space advertising.

Consider this fact: Google, the king of online marketing, is one of the top 10 direct mailers (offline) year after year. Google uses mail, newspaper, and magazine advertising, and even television and radio to drive people online. If you take a moment to examine what's happening to your mailbox every year you'll realize that it is probably getting less and less crowded. On the other hand what's happening to your email inbox and the Internet? Advertising overload.

With targeted offline advertising efforts, you can reach your ideal patients with surgeon-like precision, thus spending less to schedule a procedure than any other medium and increasing your:

- Consult capture rate
- Net scheduling rate
- Practice capture rate

In the past, I've invested significantly in creating marketing protocols for my business that revolve around both offline and online media. These protocols are part of a bag of tools that have allowed me to feel confident that every $1 I invest in marketing my business will return anywhere from $2 to more than $20 in actual sales.

When was the last time you could say that about that one-page magazine spread or the television spots you bought?

Let's get down to brass tacks. I come from a world where I have to fight it out tooth and nail with FedEx, the U.S. Postal Service (USPS), and sometimes-even UPS itself. A world where *customers begrudgingly come to my stores because they have to, not because they want to*.

On top of that, I rely on employees that have an associate degree—at best—to wait on my customers and deliver phenomenal service, all for an average sale of around $30.

In spite of this, I still went from one store to multiple stores in less than seven years in one of the most competitive marketplaces and a recession.

You, on the other hand, have clients that love you and want to come to you. They wake up in the morning and decide, "today's the day I look into plastic surgery." You will be the one who makes all of their dreams come true. And if that wasn't enough your average sale is $6,000. If I can grow my business against all odds, I can grow yours.

LOOKING AHEAD

When you create marketing protocol for your practice, you're doing two things: putting money in your bank account, and putting money in your future bank. What is a future bank you ask? It's derived from a Stephen Covey principle that states that before you launch into anything you have to "start with the end in mind."

Before you go into any medical procedure, you likely review the procedure with the members of the team assisting you and maybe even go over it in your mind. When you do this you're establishing what medical outcome you want and what steps you're going to take to achieve it.

Well, the present bank versus future bank concept is very similar to that. Before you make any decision for your practice, evaluate it by asking yourself one question, "By doing this, will it bring me patients now or will it bring me patients later?"

If the answer to that question is "no" then you simply don't do it. Marketing protocols for your practice do both. They generate patients for you know and create an asset that adds value to your practice because it can be used over and over again.

Did you think of this before you opened your practice? If the answer is "no," don't worry, I didn't do this either before I went into business.

You can fix that problem starting today.

If you think about the end now what does it look like? Do you sell your practice? Hope that a family member will be there to hand it off to? Step away from it and continue to draw income from it as a non-active shareholder? Are you going to just shut it down and ride off into the sunset? What end do you have in mind?

Your business is an asset, one that you add to and subtract from based on your actions or inactions. Creating marketing protocols adds value to your practice. They turn a traditional practice expense (marketing and advertising) into an asset.

If you knew that for every dollar you spent marketing your practice you'd get $3, $12, or even $31 back, chances are you'd jump at the opportunity to pump more money into marketing.

For many businesses—including mine—it's a reality. Let me give you an example.

Let's say there are two cosmetic practices in town—yours and a competitor's— that are identical in every apparent way. One day, they both go up for sale and one buyer is interested in buying only one of them. The buyer first meets with your competitor and reviews his financials. He finds that, while the practice's numbers are very strong, the sales price of the practice is a bit inflated. The buyer is worried that revenue levels will be impossible to maintain and wants a break on the sales price.

He then meets with you and reviews the financials of your practice. He finds that your numbers are just as strong as the other practice, but your price is 30 percent higher. Why? Because you can document how you generate those revenues with tested marketing protocols, thus reassuring the buyer that revenue levels are maintainable and even increasable if he chooses to add physicians, product lines and procedures, or even if he just raises fees.

Which practice do you think the buyer is more likely to strike a deal with in this scenario?

OTHER VALUE ADDS
Aside from adding value to your practice these protocols will also give you a better work-life balance. How?

- Automated marketing and follow-up procedures with patients.
- Patients entering the practice will be pre-sold to pay your fees.
- A shift in the patient-physician relationship from doctor to "trusted advisor."
- The ability to charge more than any other practice in town.
- The ability to see fewer patients without your current income and lifestyle being negatively affected.
- More flexibility in the type of patients you see: If you prefer "mommy makeovers," then your protocols can focus on attracting only those patients.

Perhaps the greatest benefit you will enjoy is that you will competition-proof your practice. That's right. The marketing protocols you'll employ will work so well for your practice, that, even if you revealed them to your competitors, they still wouldn't be able to compete.

So why even listen to what I have to say? Because what I'm going to share with you are tested and proven strategies that have worked for me and other business owners that I've helped.

I've got credentials, if those really matter to you. But more importantly, I've been "certified" by my real-world successes and the failures that have helped me reach those successes.

THE SCIENCE OF MARKETING

I view marketing a business as a science. It begins with a hypothesis (a marketing idea) that you want to prove true (make money with), so you set up an experiment (marketing campaign) to test it. As your experiment unfolds, you start collecting data (sales) that you then analyze to see if your hypothesis was proven or not (what was the return on your investment [ROI]).

If you collected good data, then you rerun the experiment altering a variable to test how the data changes. You repeat this process until you have optimum predictable results from your marketing protocols.

Many of the ideas I'm going to share are not new; I didn't invent them or necessarily develop them on my own. I've had a lot of help along the way. I've invested heavily in developing my skills while outsourcing to professionals the marketing components that I didn't know enough about, didn't want to do, or simply didn't have time to do. At times these investments seemed steep, but the ROI on them was immeasurable. I made the decision early on that I wasn't going to be "penny wise and dollar foolish." I surrounded myself with a team of trusted advisors to help me along the way.

The biggest discovery I made from doing this was that my greatest breakthroughs always came from people who were outside my industry, people whose opinions I would've dismissed in the early days when things were going great because I thought they couldn't possibly understand my business.

Harvard Business Review cited the study, "Integrating Problem Solvers from Analogous Markets in New Product Ideation" published by the journal *Management Science* in late 2013 in which it was revealed that, "it might pay to systematically search across firm-external sources of innovation that were formerly out of scope" and that "searching in far versus near analogous markets" provided better results. Furthermore, the study found that, "it might pay to systematically search across firm-external sources of innovation that were formerly out of scope."

MONEY BACK
GUARANTEE

This certificate entitles you to double
your money back plus $100 if you read
through the entire book and don't find
a single idea worthwhile.

To redeem this certificate
call (915) 241-7470 or fax the word
"FEFUND" on your practice letter head to
(888) 316-5887 and you will receive your
refund plus $100 within 7-10 business days.

August, 2015

DATE

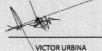

VICTOR URBINA

1

A DIFFERENT PERSPECTIVE

"Learning how to learn is life's most important skill."
— *Tony Buzan*

Where would you like your practice to be in five years? With words, paint a picture on a piece of paper that answers this question. Paint me a picture so vivid that I can smell the flowers on the reception desk, see the color of the tie you're wearing, and hear conversations of your satisfied patients in your waiting area.

If you can't answer this question with utmost detail, then in the famous words uttered from Apollo 13, "Houston, we have a problem." If you don't know where you want your practice to be in five years, then how can you realistically expect your team to help you reach your goals?

If you don't know where you want your practice to be in five years, it may be because you didn't start your practice with the end in mind.

Before long, you were so busy just doing and surviving, then growing and thriving, that you forgot all about this key step in entrepreneurship.

When you start with the end in mind, it allows you to work backwards and set up milestones that you want to hit along your journey. These milestones will keep you on track and help you reach your ultimate goal.

A captain of a ship doesn't set sail from a harbor blindly, not knowing what his final destination will be and the best route for reaching it. He plans his course, checks his progress along the way, and makes adjustments whenever he's deviated direction. The famous plastic surgeon and "Psycho-Cybernetics" author Maxwell Maltz, stated that we all have an automatic, self-correcting mechanism inside of us that puts us back on course whenever we stray too far from our intended target. When you do this for your practice, it provides you with rules that you can abide by in order to reach your goal. Starting with the end in mind dictates expansion plans, hiring practices, product line or procedure additions, and even how much time off you take.

If you're not operating with the end in mind, don't worry. Your course can be corrected and your destination can be altered. If you start now, you will still reach a desirable destination; your voyage can still be salvaged.

YOUR NEW PRACTICE

Your practice is your biggest asset and one that, unfortunately, keeps its full value locked inside of it until the day you decide to sell.

Everything you do has a positive or negative impact on the bottom line. Did you just hire a new receptionist that chews gum loudly when she answers the phone? That's going to cost you more than just her salary. Are you reaching out to past patients and just checking in with them every two or three months? If you are, congratulations, you're making deposits in your future bank.

You know that you have to invest in your practice if you want to cash out handsomely. You will recuperate a percentage of every dollar you invest in your practice at the end of the day.

But what if I told you that there are certain investments in your business that will return multiples of the amount invested, not a percentage of it? Would you invest more aggressively in these areas that are guaranteed to give you outcomes beyond anything else?

Welcome to your "new" practice. Imagine starting every month knowing what your billings will be. Imagine being able to block off entire weeks from your calendar to spend time with your friends and family or for that extended trip to Europe you've been wanting to take, but have put off because you'll lose prospective patients to competitors. Imagine coming home in time for dinner, being able to pick up your kids from school, or being able to take the afternoons off so you can go to your daughter's soccer game without worrying about your practice. *Imagine being mentally present* when you're with your family and friends!

Creating marketing protocols will allow you the flexibility to introduce new product lines and procedures without the uncertainty of whether or not they will succeed. You will be able to collect market data prior to a launch with the protocols you developed to gauge demand. Once you have established that there is an acceptable level of demand, you will already have your marketing tactics in place to go out and capture those patients.

The beauty of marketing protocols is that they can be adapted to any market, any product, at any time. You don't need to reinvent the wheel every time you launch something new; just take one of your successful campaigns of the shelf, dust it off, and update it to make it relevant to what you're promoting.

Remember, a buyer is a buyer is a buyer, and once you're able to crack the code and attract the best ones to your practice, you'll be able to put aspects of your practice on autopilot.

The #1 frustration that all business owners face is not enough customers. If you analyze why they don't have enough customers you'll probably find one of two things:

- NO marketing, or
- BAD marketing

What would your life be like if you could eliminate this frustration from it?

Running a close second to not having enough customers is the frustration of not enough time. Wouldn't it be great if you could have more free time without your income suffering? If you are the sole surgeon in your practice, then the income your practice generates correlates to the number of hours you put in. That weight is entirely on your shoulders.

Maybe you have a practice manager who helps you with the administrative side, and they might even be pulling double duty as your marketing manager. You and I both know that they are overworked and stressed out by the workload, and it's likely that one of the two roles is suffering and costing you money.

Establishing protocols in your practice will eliminate the burden and allow you to hang on to your superstar staff without experiencing burnout. It's well-known that salespeople don't get burned out from selling, they get burned out from prospecting.

Without tested, proven, repeatable, and profitable marketing protocols in place for your practice, you are in essence "prospecting" every time you advertise. The "prospecting" continues when you put prospective patients in front of your treatment coordinator to close the sale. Repeated iterations of this with poor or no measurable results eventually lead to burnout and sometimes cause practices to swear off advertising and marketing altogether. Systematizing your practice and developing protocols allows you to have less stress and more free time to decompress, and ensures the financial future of your practice.

WHAT ABOUT COMPETITION?

I say the more the merrier, because they are helping create awareness and demand for the services you provide and your practice, with its superior marketing protocols, will capitalize on this.

Look, I'm not going to lie to you, the marketing you're going to be doing is complex, time-consuming to set up, and different than what you're accustomed to. You are going to be investing smartly every month marketing your practice. You're going to use tactics that have demonstrated that they have earned their share of your money; they will have measurable, verifiable, and repeatable returns on investment of every dollar you spend.

Your competition, well, they'll be like chum in the water, helping attract the big fish. You practice will have the best bait and will be the one with the winning catch, time after time. I'm not talking about netting all the customers; you're not going to catch every one that swims by. You *will* catch the best in the sea of customers; the ones that will like and respect you and be presold on doing business with you before they even show up for their initial consultation.

No more free initial consults. Your patients are going to be eager and willing to pay any fee to get in your door. Your marketing is going to do as much to attract quality patients, as it will to repel the wrong patients for your practice.

What is that worth to you? Working only with patients that are eager to meet with you, will follow all your instructions, will not shop you, and most importantly, that will become your raving fans and proselytize others for you?

As I said before you're marketing is going to be complex and different. It will be so complex that, even if you gave your competitors specific instructions for how to do it, they won't follow in your footsteps. Why? Well because, upfront, it takes a little work. This is not a get-rich-quick scheme promising to make you millions overnight. I'm not a metaphysical guru telling you that if you focus on new patient attraction long enough customers will magically appear.

I think we can both agree that you didn't get to this position in life by focusing on the "white light" emanating from something and then it magically appearing. Nope, you've busted your butt and know that that's what it really takes to be successful, that without a little pain there's never any real gain. This is exactly what your competition is not willing to do.

I'm not saying they don't work hard. What I'm saying is that they are not actively looking to bring complexity into their practice. Most are just following the herd.

When mall banners advertising your practice became the "shiny new button" all practices just had to have, what did everyone do? They all went out and paid for one. Maybe you did, too, or if you didn't, it's only because someone else bought it out from under you. In other words, your competitors were more willing to take wads of cash out of their bank account, stack it neatly in a pile, pour some gasoline on it, strike a match, and light it on fire.

I'm not saying that mall banners don't work, they do, and they can work very well, but without an adequate plan behind this tactic that includes measurement of outcomes, it's all a waste.

So, yes, your marketing is going to get complex and eventually it will take some time to set up, but business is a complex animal, and your practice is no different than any other business. *We are all the same.* Customers with money come in one end, and customers having partaken of your product or service go out the other end.

WHY PEOPLE BUY

People all buy things for the same reasons: They have a void that needs to be filled. For most, that void is an emotional one.

Very few people can tell you with a high degree of certainty the exact logical reason why they purchase anything. If you ask they will probably give one or two customary answers: "The deal was too good to pass up!" "I needed it!" etc. Those reasons might be true, but they don't tell us the real reason why, you would have to dig a little deeper and ask a few questions to find out. That is of course assuming a buyer could enunciate, beyond these superficial reasons, why they bought.

They key to successful patient attraction is being able to tap into this void and provide your services as a possible solution.

If you can enter the conversation that's already going on in your prospective patients' heads, then they will see your practice as an ideal fit for them.

Even better if you could create the conversation in their heads, then your practice would be on a whole other level and become almost untouchable; patients would see no other practice on their radar because yours is so well aligned with them.

Why would you even want to do anything like this? Well because when you enter or even create the conversation going on in your patient's head you change the whole game. You can set the buying criteria. The level or expertise they should look for when interviewing physician. Even the features and benefits to expect from a practice. Your message will be so congruent with how they see themselves that they will have no logical reason to go to anyone else.

Congruence is important because it is highly linked to how we make decisions, often times forcing us to choose something not to our benefit in order to remain congruent with how we see ourselves. It's the primary reason political parties want you to "declare" your party of affiliation as early as possible. They know that once you've "declared" yourself for a specific party you will vote for that party almost regardless of the candidates. It's the secret behind "straight ticket" voting.

So as you can see congruence is very important in how we make decisions and the reason why you want to enter or create the conversation in a patient's head. You want them to see your practice as congruent with how they see themselves.

A NEGATIVE SNOWBALL EFFECT

Is your net scheduling rate what you would like it to be every month? If it is, are they the type of procedures that you enjoy most? If it's stacked with procedures you dread, it's because you're attracting the wrong type of patients. If you don't have enough every month it's because patients are shopping you after they visit your office and you're not closing the consultations, or because your marketing isn't working and you don't have enough initial consultations — plain and simple.

When the above scenarios happen, a negative snowball effect happens:

- You're more stressed at work and at home because of the financial uncertainty of your practice.
- You become irritable to your staff and appear desperate in front of patients.
- You start to negotiate on your pricing in order to land more patients and include more post-op freebies.

Heaven forbid you start to haggle over pricing with a patient; that is acting more like a car salesman than a medical professional. If you or your treatment coordinator are already doing this, then you didn't do a good enough job leading up to the consultation. You didn't create any authority for your practice, you didn't create any celebrity, and you didn't establish yourself as the go-to expert. When you haggle over pricing, you're arguing with your patient. You may not have realized this, but the sales process with that patient began way before your receptionist picked up the phone and scheduled them for a consultation.

If you start negotiating your fees, before you know it, you have to schedule more and more procedures to cover your practice expenses and maintain your current lifestyle. If you have a line of credit for your practice, you start dipping into it a little more and a little more to offset declining revenues.

Let's face it: Even though you're now working like a dog and are a slave to your practice there's only so much you can do in a day. If you have to increase your current workload by only 5 to 10 percent, how many additional hours would that be every month? Good thing everything is still going smoothly at home, right? Or is your spouse already complaining that you're never home in time to eat dinner as a family. Your kids don't know you and you feel like you have to put on a nametag the minute you walk in the door. Worst of all, you still haven't found a way to tell them that you might have to cancel one of your scheduled vacations because money is tight right now.

If any of these statements sound familiar, welcome to the club. I have been there done that, I feel your pain.

What's worse is that everyone sees you as a great success, when in reality, you're just surviving and the house of cards can all come crashing down any minute. Again, I understand your pain.

BUSINESS IS BUSINESS

There are a lot of commonalities between a retail business and a cosmetic practice. The biggest one is that we are not selling a product or service, we're selling the transformation.

In cosmetic practices, this is easier to understand than in a traditional business, but the fact still remains. As Harvard Business School marketing professor Theodore Levitt said, "People don't want to buy a quarter-inch drill. They want a quarter-inch hole." People come into my UPS Stores not to ship something; they come in because they want to surprise their 10-year-old grandson across the country with a special gift on his birthday.

So we are both selling a transformation of some sort. That transformation could also be filling a void a patient has inside of them. Maybe it's low or nonexistent self-confidence in social situations, maybe it's being self-conscious about a scar or birthmark they have on their face, or maybe it's much deeper and involves a complete makeover after a traumatic life event. Again, we sell the transformation not the product.

Perhaps the biggest commonality is that, like all businesses, we all rely on a steady stream of customers. Whether they are new or repeat doesn't matter, although it is significantly cheaper and easier to sell more to your existing patients that it is to attract new ones. We'll talk about that later. Without the ability to consistently and affordably attract customers to our business we're doomed. Nothing happens until someone enters my stores or your office; until then, all we have a very expensive hobby.

I struggled with customer attraction myself. I would spend thousands of dollars every month running radio ads, discounting services (coupons), and sending out postcards without a clue as to whether they were actually working. I couldn't for the life of me tell you what the return on investment (ROI) was on our marketing investment.

It goes without saying that all businesses need a good reputation. People need to trust that when they walk into one of my stores, my associates will package their shipment as if it were their own. They need to trust that we will not make a mistake in the address when we label their package. Most importantly they need to trust that UPS will deliver their package safely and on time.

Those are the basic deliverables and expectations of our transactions; I'm sure they are not that different from yours. Patients expect that you will care for them pre- and post-op as if they were a part of your own family. They trust that you won't make mistakes during the procedure. Most importantly they trust that you will do everything within your power to ensure that they have a positive outcome with a speedy and full recovery. Those are your deliverables and expectations.

If we fail with even one of these deliverables, our reputation is definitely tarnished with that customer or patient, sometimes irreparably. Did you know that a customer that has a negative experience with you is likely to tell up to 10 more people about that experience than one who has had a positive one? This is true in any line of work.

Lastly, we both need our businesses to be profitable. Let's face it: We both got into business to make as much money as we could, in the shortest amount of time, with the least amount of work possible. There's nothing wrong with admitting that we're both capitalists that want to be part of the 1 percent. It's the reason we both studied for as long as we did, that we work as hard as we do, and that we have sacrificed as much as we have. Just think of how many of these activities you've missed: birthdays, vacations, nights out with friends, family get-togethers, a good night's sleep.

Yet, I consider building as much wealth as I possibly can an integral part of my life's goal, and you should, too. It will allow you to give to people and causes that you consider important without the expectation of getting something back. It will ensure the financial future of your entire family, possibly for generations to come.

The biggest thing that money can buy is autonomy, allowing you to march to the beat of your own drum, live life on your terms, and conduct your business the way you want to, not the way everyone expects you to. In a sentence, *"To have the world revolve around you!"*

Along with autonomy and money come options. Wealthy people have options in everything they do from what they eat for breakfast to the quality of medical care they receive. In short, having options is a pretty sweet deal. We can't have options and we can't have autonomy if our business isn't profitable.

THE IMPORTANCE OF ROI

Beyond profitability, our business needs to have positive cash flow. Cash is what pays the bills and keeps our business alive. It's what's left after you've paid all your bills and operating expenses. It's not the top-line number you might refer to as sales or billings. You can have huge billings every month, but if you don't cover your expenses you will slowly put yourself out of business. It's like having a bucket full of water with a hole in it—slowly all the water will leak out of it.

Let me give you a real life example to illustrate how important ROI is in a business from my own experiences. A while back I was analyzing buying another UPS Store in a different part of the country. The owner needed to sell the business for numerous reasons and had set what I considered a high sales price, so I asked for financial information on the business to perform my due diligence. Upon inspection of the financials it was obvious to me that the business wasn't worth even 10 percent of the asking price.

I made my concerns known to the seller and asked for an explanation on how he reached his sales price. He said the number he came up with was based on the business being set up to generate sales of over $1 million in the future.

To be honest, I was a bit shocked by this answer. I had never heard of a business selling based solely on speculated sales figures without verification of how those numbers would be reached. I know all businesses have a certain amount of "goodwill" attached to their value, but this was bordering on the absurd.

I made the business owner an offer based on a multiple of his current net income, minus a 20 percent sales premium because I knew for a fact that the owner of the business was the principal sales driver. There were no guarantees that the personal relationships and contacts he had developed over the years would remain intact after he stepped out of the business. Goodwill is a very subjective thing; there is no hard line item on a balance sheet showing an exact figure. In this case, the business' "goodwill" acted against the business.

To make a long story short, we were miles apart on a deal and we never struck one. It was a solid business that could be profitable, but the owner's unrealistic valuation and dependence on its "goodwill" were huge obstacles that we couldn't overcome.

What if, instead, the owner had shown me that he had established systems for generating sales? If he had paraded out a series of marketing campaigns he uses throughout the year with measurable and verifiable results that were predictable. If he had shown me that those same campaigns had generated increased sales year to year, and he based his sales price on those sales projections, then I would've had a much easier time accepting his valuation. It probably would've left me very little room—if any—to try and negotiate a discount of any sort on the sales prices. The argument of "goodwill," while still important to a business, would've been a nonissue. The business owner wouldn't have needed it because he had protocols in place that drove revenue, not the whim of the market.

This, my friend, is why I've created protocols for all my businesses, and I encourage you to do the same. I plan on cashing out one day and I would rather step into those negotiations knowing that my sales price is fair and justifiable and that I don't have to defend it. Wouldn't you like to do the same?

THE 10/10/80 PHENOMENON

As I've said before: A buyer is a buyer is a buyer. People all buy for the exact same reasons. They have an unfulfilled need that they're trying to fill.

The old adage "nature abhors a vacuum, and it will do whatever it takes to fill it," can be said of consumers. They will fill a vacuum with anything they think will help fill it—why not your services?

Marketing is a numbers game. Studies have shown that at any given time if you fill a room with 100 people, and you're selling any product or service, 10 of them are ready to buy and will buy—right then and there. Another 10 of those people will never buy from you for any number of reasons; maybe they just bought what you're selling, maybe they don't like your product, or maybe their brother sells the exact same thing. That leaves 80 people in the room with some level of interest in what you're selling—they haven't said no to your product, so they're "listening." I call this the 10/10/80 phenomenon.

What do you do to capitalize on these 80 people? You paid to get into this room and you paid to reach all 100 people; why are you walking away satisfied after only selling to a few of the 10 that were ready to buy (because, come on, you're not going to sell to all 10)? Wouldn't it be smart to do something about the other 80?

The minute I understood this, I realized I was leaving a lot of money on the table by only focusing on the 10 that are ready to buy now. I realized that with a little time and effort, I could possibly get an additional 10 to 30 to buy, given a sufficient amount of time. It forced me to completely restructure the way I was marketing my business.

Let's talk about another consumer behavior that I'm sure you love and that we're all guilty of—shopping!

Before consumers buy just about anything these days, they shop, research, read reviews, ask friends, etc. Wouldn't it be smart if you could bypass all of this with your ideal patients? The affluent market, the one that you are after, relies more on recommendations from friends and family than anything you could ever advertise to them.

You see, what happens when someone is looking for a plastic surgeon, because they're thinking about rhinoplasty or any other procedure, is they often look online. What happened the last time you went searching for a product to buy online? Did you stop shopping once you found it? Did you keep looking to see what else was out there in an effort to find it cheaper or with free shipping? You compared businesses, or in this case websites, right?

Guess what: Your customers are doing the same thing to you. They're shopping you, comparing you. Many don't care how many certifications you have on your wall or what awards you've won; *for them, price rules*.

Recall what your journey was like the last time you discovered something new that you really wanted. Was it a great author or band? A great pair of pants? An awesome vacation spot? Did you research that specific thing obsessively like a lunatic? My guess is you did, and no matter what other, similar options presented themselves to you, they didn't quite live up to the genuine article, right? You found reasons why they were inferior.

You see, we all make buying decisions emotionally, but then we use logic to justify those decisions. When the brain is consumed with emotion it has no room to think logically. It's been proven, most recently by Raj Raghunathan marketing professor at the McCombs School of Business in a study that asked participants to choose between an attractive chicken and an ugly chicken. Let's face it our reptilian brains can still only handle one train of thought or emotion at a time.

Think about it for a second. The last time you bought a car, what did the salesperson do? He tried to become your friend, to get you laughing, to get you to make small commitments to buying a car or taking it for a test drive. Before you knew it, you were sitting in the finance office forking over a check for 20 percent and agreeing to all kinds of things that weren't in your favor. Why? Because your logical mind didn't have a chance to get a word in, you were consumed with the feeling of euphoria and excitement.

It's a little like that for people attracted to your practice. They all go through three pre-purchase and two post-purchase stages. They start off as "suspects," which are people that you suspect would be interested in a cosmetic procedure, but they have done nothing to indicate they would. Your suspicion is based strictly on your own first-hand experience.

Suspects become leads once they express an interest in you, your practice, or a particular procedure. They, in essence, raise their hands and tell you, "I want to learn more."

At this point the "courting" process begins and they become a prospect. It is your responsibility to educate this prospect and help them make the best decision about what they want to purchase, which ultimately should be your services. The goal during the entire prospect phase is to get them into your practice for a consultation.

Once they are in your practice and you've closed the appointment, the prospect becomes a patient—but that's not the end of the journey. You have to ensure that you continue educating these patients and further developing your relationship with them so that you can reach the final stage.

That final stage is to convert these patients into clients. Clients are a step above patients because you only need one transaction to generate a patient. Clients on the other hand are those patients that return two or three times a year and refer their friends to your practice. The goal of your practice, and any business for that matter, is to create clients.

THE TRANSFORMATION
I've tried many, many methods to get to where I am today with the

marketing of my business. Some have been superstars and some, well, not so much. If I had to give myself a batting average, I'd say I'm batting about .300; so one out of every three things I've tried have worked. Would I love to have all winners? Absolutely, but that's not realistic, and anyone who guarantees you that is lying to you.

In fact, I had a number of losers before I got my first winner; that first big win was a pretty straightforward campaign targeted at our existing customers. It had been active for about five months before we got our first really measureable hit —and it was a big one! That campaign brought in a sale that shot up its ROI to almost $30 for every $1 that I had invested on it to that point. I couldn't invest money in it fast enough the next month. I would've never gotten to that point had I not been diligently tracking what I was doing and measuring the outcomes to weed out the bad ideas and keep the superstars.

Let me give you another example. I launched another campaign for the holidays last year. As you might imagine, the holiday season is a very busy time for a UPS Store. People ship gifts all over the country; you might've even done it yourself.

Well, we ran a campaign that delivered an ROI of about $1.76 for every $1 that I invested. It didn't set the world on fire, but it definitely earned its keep.

More importantly, it brought in customers we didn't see the year before and it allowed me to communicate with all of this year. So the true ROI of this campaign hasn't really been completely measured. Next, we're going to take this same campaign and trot it out during the non-holiday season, make some tweaks to it, and see how it performs. A buyer is a buyer is a buyer right? Well, we will have to measure and see.

The point I'm trying to make is that you can't be afraid to try new things. If you have something that's working, test it to see if you can have it perform better. You'll never know just how much money you might be leaving on the table until you test.

So how did I wind up writing this book and helping cosmetic plastic surgeons? Well, because your business deals with transformations, and I saw a huge gap in how you market your practices. Currently, most of your marketing efforts are probably online, and most marketers will tell you that this is the most viable means of marketing your practice. Those people do amazing work and they are very knowledgeable about what they do, but as I've mentioned before, what happens when someone is searching for you online? Do they stop after they've found your website or seen your video? Nope, they're in "shopping mode." They don't necessarily want to shop on price, but most of the time you've given them no other way to compare two seemingly identical practices!

I'm going to teach you how to fill that gap, how to be "discovered." I'm going to show you how to control more of the information your "suspects" see, and to create a much stronger bond between you and them before they even book an appointment and set foot in your practice. Remember selling doesn't start when a patient schedules a consultation.

Here's the twist: This is going to be done offline! That's right, through good old-fashioned newspaper and magazine advertising, inserts, and dare I say—direct mail.

HOW A COSMETIC SURGERY PRACTICE IS LIKE A RETAIL STORE

- Both depend on a steady stream of new and repeat customers or patients.
- Both sell transformations.
- Both are susceptible to being "shopped" by customers and patients.
- Reputation is everything to both.
- Cash is king, it takes positive cash flows to keep both afloat.
- Measurable marketing ROI is the only tool both have to justify any spend.
- Both have to make payroll every other week.
- Both become very philanthropic once a certain level of success is achieved.

2

WHY CURRENT MARKETING
EFFORTS AREN'T ENOUGH

"There is only one boss. The customer.
And he can fire everybody in the company
from the chairman on down,
simply by spending his money somewhere else."
– Sam Walton

Currently if I were to look to through any of your existing marketing pieces, I'll bet they would look like all of your competitors. In fact, if I were to pull pieces from different practices all over the country, yours may be almost identical to someone else's. How do you expect a suspect to differentiate between you and your competitors and compare you based on anything other than fee when everything you're putting in front of them looks the same?

You probably have a pretty girl in your ad and copy that touts "letting your inner beauty out" or something like "the look you've always dreamed of." Wow, that's super original! Did the art department for the agency that sold you the ad come up with that line and you just nod dumbly in agreement?

However, the biggest mistake you're probably making with your marketing is a weak or nonexistent offer. Offers like "Free consultation" or "Breast augmentation starting at $999" aren't very strong offers.

This goes back to the 10/10/80 phenomenon we discussed in the previous chapter. These offers capitalize almost exclusively on the low-hanging fruit, the 10 percent that are ready to buy now.

The thing is that you're vying for this 10 percent of your market with all your competition. So again, when a suspect that doesn't know any better starts to "shop" for a procedure or service guess what criterion she's going to use to make her buying decision? Price.

Sure, having a nice office and being centrally located will influence the buying decision to some degree, but with all things being equal—and unless the lowest fee in town is a disreputable dump—the buyer is going to choose the cheapest or the second cheapest chicken, because we've all been taught to never buy the cheapest because there's probably something wrong with it.

The next thing to understand is that you're only giving people one way of responding to your offer and there is a huge barrier to response for a suspect that is still in the exploratory phase.

Think about the last time you bought a car: Did you head straight to a dealership for a test drive? I'm guessing you didn't, very few of us would.

Instead, you probably researched online, narrowed your field down to two or three choices, possibly spoke to other owners of the same models, and then headed to the dealership for a test drive.

What you're asking your suspects to do by coming in for a free consultation is the equivalent of heading straight to a dealership without first doing any sort of research. Very few people are going to do that.

Do you really want to do **free consults**? It's a waste of your time and **attracts all the wrong prospects**. It positions you just like everyone else in town that's doing free consults. It **undervalues your time** in the eyes of a prospect and lowers their respect for your expertise. How much **did you care about the last thing you got for free?** Done right, **the initial consult should act to repel as much as it does to attract** ideal patients. Patients that are going to like and respect you, your time, and your practice. **Free is the wrong way to start.**

What if you made your suspects an offer that appeals to the 10 percent that are ready to buy now, and if you gave the remaining 80 percent a method of gathering more information about the procedure and your practice without them having to stroll into your office? Maybe you're already sending them to your website to watch videos. That's a good first step, but what good is it to have a website with a lot of traffic if you don't know how well it's converting? I don't know about you, but I can't deposit website traffic in the bank and it's not because I didn't try, believe me.

Your Web designer or marketing director probably loves pointing to all these stats—how many hits, average site-visit duration, search terms that brought them to your site, etc. They're oblivious to the fact that all these stats don't mean squat if you can correlate them directly to scheduled procedures.

Look, it's very simple, the website you send suspects to has one job and one job only—to capture a suspect's information and convert her to a lead. Period! Your website should be a lead-capture tool. It doesn't need tabs, links, a Facebook "like" button. It needs to have a way to offer information in exchange for the suspects' information. You can have your main page isolated from the landing page that you give out to people after you've captured their information, *but not before*. What you're trying to do is eliminate their options on your lead capture site and control the conversation you want to have with them.

So back to my car example: A controlled landing page would be the equivalent of looking at brochures, reports, videos, etc. on a website or sites, except you've captured a suspect's information and converted her to a lead.

My last comment about offers: Rarely do I see a deadline associated with them. *An offer without some sort of deadline is not an offer, it's a statement.* You need to give people a reason to act now. Any of these types of deadlines will do in your offers:

- Limited time.
- Limited quantity.
- Bonus with purchase.

Always have a deadline and be sure you communicate that in all your marketing.

IMAGE AND BRAND

Let's talk about image and brand. Marketers today love to talk about brand: "you need to build your brand," "you have to brand yourself," "think about your brand." Well, I hate to burst your bubble, but unless you're Nike or Coca Cola or Mercedes-Benz, nobody is going to care about your brand. Why should they? Who do you think you are, a Kardashian? They don't know you from Adam. People don't care about you, until you give them a reason to, and they know how much you care.

Do you understand that statement? Read it again and let it sink in. People don't care about you, until you give them a reason to, and they know how much you care.

How do you show a prospective or even a suspect patient how much you care? One way of doing this is by educating them on the investment they're about to make with no strings attached. When you do this, you're really doing a great service to not only your patient, but to your entire profession because it force other practices to "step their game up" because they know they're dealing with a sophisticated buyer. It will force the charlatans to either shape up or ship out.

It also changes the way you're perceived by a patient. It turns you into a trusted advisor, a "consigliere." I've seen this strategy work so successfully that it virtually melts away all apprehension a patient might have over fees because they understand the true value of what they're getting.

When a patient knows how much you care, then and only then will they proselytize for you and thus you begin to build your "brand."

If you're not doing this and you're going to market your business based solely on brand, you're committing a huge mistake. You're going to spend literally tens of thousands of dollars trying to build your brand before you even put a dent in peoples' consciousness about who you are.

This is not to say that brand isn't important, but you can build your brand while at the same time achieving measurable positive outcomes from your marketing protocols.

Most marketing consultants really have no skin in the game. They work for an agency or they're solo-preneurs who have never had to make payroll every other Friday like us. Many of them are double-dipping or moonlighting.

Here's an "inside baseball" tip: If you're letting your outside marketing rep do all your media buys for you and then invoicing you or giving you an all-inclusive quote, they're probably padding the actual price by anywhere from 5 to 15 percent. This is a pretty standard practice. You should always ask for original invoices from media providers so you can pay them directly or at least keep your marketing rep honest.

THE A.C.E. PRINCIPLE

So how do you build your brand while at the same time building your practice? The number one way I recommend you do this is by setting yourself apart from your competitors by using the A.C.E. principle. This stands for authority, celebrity, and exclusivity. When done successfully, this can be transferred to your practice and become almost independent of who the actual surgeons are. Instead, the practice itself is what becomes well known.

This will allow you to fetch a premium price not only for your services, but also from a potential buyer if and when you decide to sell your practice.

Let's talk about the different components of the principle.

First, the A, which stands for authority. How are you positioning yourself and your practice to be the authority in your market? You can do this any number of ways, but the method I recommend is that you niche. In other words, become a specialist in a particular procedure; don't be a generalist. Look at your own profession. Who makes more money, a neurosurgeon or a general practitioner?

I'm not saying you wipe everything else off the menu either. What I'm saying is find one procedure that has the most potential in your market — maybe it's facelifts because there are a lot of affluent boomers in your community — and then market specifically to that segment. For example, include the phrase "specializing in facelifts for women over 50 in Orange County." You see what I did with that one sentence? I immediately called out exactly who my services were for, I created affinity with my suspects over my competitors who are just advertising "facelifts starting at $2,000." and I made a potential lead see herself or an acquaintance as someone who fits the bill.

Hand in hand with authority comes the C of the principle, which stands for celebrity. Once people know you are the local authority on a certain procedure, you could put out reports, buying guides, and educational videos; hold seminars; or even author a book — all aimed at your ideal prospect to further heighten your authority and celebrity.

The last piece of the principle is the E, which stands for exclusivity. What you do here is very simple, you raise your fees and you limit access to you. In a word, you become exclusive. If possible, start a waiting list. Make it challenging for patients to even get that first paid consultation with you. If you understand how this works, you'll realize that this is no different than what country clubs, luxury automakers, and even the top restaurants in the country do. Everyone wants to be part of the exclusive "insider" crowd; dining frequently at an exclusive restaurant or golfing regularly at an exclusive country club makes you feel special. Guess what? You probably tell your friends and relatives all about it. In doing so, you're promoting the business that made you jump through hoops in order for you to do business with it. Does that seem a little counterintuitive? Sure it does, but when your practice has the mojo and is the place to go you'll be glad our primate brains are as dysfunctional as they are.

People will buy from you for only four reasons: price, service, quality, and exclusivity. All things being equal, I would much rather be on the exclusive end of that spectrum.

BEING TARGETED AND SPECIFIC

When you're first starting and wanting to establish your authority, you'll want to be as targeted and specific as possible, so you need to speak directly to your prospects' pain points. Every "we" statement (or the features your practice offers) in your marketing should also include a "you" statement (which are the benefits your patients derive from your services).

When you speak to your prospects' specific pain points you can then speak to them about how your services will provide the transformation they're looking for. People will "buy what you're selling" more readily if you think like they do. (Think: What's in it for me?)

If you're still working on being the authority, consider what authorities do. They educate.

Educate your consumer on the specific procedure they're considering. Now I'm not talking about textbook diagrams or taking them through an anatomy lesson. Educate them about yourself and your practice. Sure, you're going to tell them about the procedure, but without being clinical.

What are you talking about? The transformation!

I don't propose strictly using testimonials either, it's much deeper than that. Talk about how other patients identical to them came to you and how you've changed their lives. Explain how they are now more confident in social situations, how they rekindled their romance with their spouse, how they reclaimed the vitality that was inside them all along.

Then ask them to request more information via a low-barrier method in order to get them to step forward and identify themselves to you as being interested in the transformation. You can then follow up with them, continuing to educate them until one of two things happens: Either they step forward and say I'm ready, at which point they make a paid appointment, or they no longer qualify as viable prospects, at which point you still continue to follow up with them, but not as frequently.

In order to make any type of sale you have to tell a prospect what's in it for them. Prospects don't care that you're the best at what you do, up to this point, why should they? Why should anyone? If your marketing is all about "we" and "I" then you're doing it wrong. You're trying to sell exclusively based on features, just like all of your competitors.

You need to focus on the benefits your patients will enjoy. Remember: You're selling the hole not the drill. So your marketing needs to be loaded with benefits instead of features. It needs to speak to your prospect directly, almost as if you're writing them a personal letter and they're a dear friend.

That's actually a great exercise: Write a letter to yourself in the voice of your ideal patient. What would they write to you about? Once you have it written, then mail it to yourself. You'll find that when you get the letter in the mail a few days later it'll have a much deeper impact on you versus just reading it in your office fresh after writing it.

Once you've read and truly understand the letter's contents, focus your marketing on solving the pain points the patient expressed in your letter. This will get you thinking more about benefits instead of features.

BUYING BEHAVIOR AND ONLINE MARKETING

Let's have a little talk about how many people buy at any given moment. If I were to walk into your office where you employ 10 people, and I had a great pizza offer, I would sell one pizza almost immediately upon entering. On the flip side of that, there would be one person in your office who would tell me, they hate pizza, they're on a diet, or their husband makes the best homemade brick oven pizza in the world. They are never going to buy my pizza. That leaves eight people in your office who still have varying levels of interest in pizza.

A salesperson who is not very bright would smile on his good fortune of having made one easy sale and quickly thanked you and exited your office. He'll feast his whole career on low-hanging fruit sales (or in this case, pizza), knocking on twice as many doors to sell less than what he could, and in the process burning out.

A smart salesman, however, would take the contact information for the remaining eight people in your office and continue to follow up with them until his offer ends. He'll find that, along the way, he'll generate two to four more sales and one referral from his efforts. He generated five times more sales from that one encounter than the bad salesman and saved four times as much time. This is how you have to think about your marketing.

A lot of cosmetic practice marketing gurus preach the value of online marketing. They do this for three reasons:

- They don't know any better and are attracted to the "glittering object" in the marketing world.
- They like the idea that it's "cheap," therefore you can do a lot of it.
- They have no understanding of consumer buying behavior.

When you focus exclusively online, you're opening Pandora's Box. You're putting your practice out there to be compared, to be shopped. So you're going to be compared to other practices based on the one thing that a customer can grasp to compare—price.

Let me expand on this discussion from the previous chapter.

When people shop for something online, very rarely do they stop after finding what they need. The majority of the time they continue to shop for options. They may be looking for a different color, different features, free delivery maybe, and of course a cheaper price. This is basic consumer behavior, and it's often based on the fact that they don't know enough about what they're looking for to be able to compare two seemingly identical options by any other method.

When you market exclusively online you commoditize your practice, making it interchangeable with any other practice in town. You really don't differentiate it in any way, and you have to sell exclusively on price. It's a race to the bottom; he who charges the lowest price will win the majority of the business. When you capitalize on all the low-hanging fruit in a market, you eventually run out of patients. In the future, you have to spend more and more to reach new low-hanging fruit because all your competitors are doing the same thing. Again, before you know it, you're working 12 to 14 hours a day to earn the same or less than you did only a year or two ago.

How different do you think the above scenario would be if your patients instead "discovered" you? Do you think that the selling process would be different? Absolutely.

Whenever we discover something, we want to research more about the topic almost immediately. We develop an insatiable thirst to learn.

Why not give the public what it wants?

TARGETING YOUR EFFORTS

Let me expand on what I mean by "discover."

Once upon a time, our mailboxes were littered with direct mail flyers—

cards, leaflets, letters, all asking us to buy, buy, buy.

Now, the Internet has become our mailbox. Every year, our physical mailboxes get less and less cluttered, and our email inboxes get more and more crowded.

By going back to the traditional method of communication, you'll find there is less competition and less clutter to cut through to grab a suspect's attention. If you speak to your ideal patient's specific pain points in your offline marketing, focus on the transformation, give them a low-commitment way request more information, and educate them in the process, then you will be more successful than your competition.

But it's a huge expectation for any type of marketing to make a life-changing sale like cosmetic plastic surgery on its own; even the best salesperson would see that task as difficult at best. So don't ask your marketing to do all the heavy lifting.

Instead, use your marketing efforts to get incremental commitments from suspect patients. Once a suspect requests more information, she officially becomes a lead and you can begin the education and selling process.

At that point, you're essentially bringing your leads into a room and closing the door behind them. You will have complete control over what kind of information they receive. You will decide who can enter and when they can leave the room. You will even decide if they see your competitor's ads.

By controlling the information and ads your leads receive, you're positioning your practice to be the authority and the celebrity in your market, making you the only logical choice for them. Why would they go anywhere else?

Up until this point, you've probably been doing a lot of "spraying and praying" with your practices marketing. Even those practices that have a "marketing manager," are often only using someone on the office staff—who already has a full plate—to do their marketing efforts. If you are using "spraying and praying," then there's likely no way you can measure the ROI on the marketing tactic you used. At best, you might be able to say "we got some calls," "sales went up," or more likely, "it didn't work."

So let's look at each of those responses for a minute.

First, "we got some calls." Fantastic! How do you know they were in response to your offer? Was it a unique ad-only offer or one they could get at any time? Did you use some sort of tracking number or tracking code to assign a hit to that campaign? Did you at least ask the callers how they heard of you?

Next, "sales went up." Also fantastic! Now, can you accurately attribute an increase in sales to your tactic? Again, did you run ad-specific offers? Did you have a way for tracking responses? If you ran multiple tactics, was each one unique? What did you measure that helped you determine that your tactics was why sales went up?

Finally, "it didn't work." Really? How are you so sure? Did you ask all your leads or patients how they heard about your practice? Did you have a method for tracking in your tactic?

Again, unless you're measuring your marketing efforts, you won't really know what works and what doesn't. If you're measuring, you can calculate the ROI on a tactic and objectively determine if it can stay in the rotation and be altered or if it's a tactic that needs to be retired from your arsenal.

Marketing is the most important component of you practice. Would you pay an employee at your practice to do a very specific, crucial job and then allow her to show up to work only two or three times a month? Then why do you do this with your marketing?

Everything you do to market your practice has to earn its keep. When you do this you take what your competitors consider to be an expense and turn it into an asset — a verifiable and real asset that adds value to your practice.

When you see your successes, you will be eager to invest.

Notice that I said "invest," because whenever we invest in something, we do it with the expectation of receiving a return greater than or at least equal to our initial investment. Once you see marketing as an investment, you're going to stop "spending" on advertising. There's a difference between "investing" and "spending." We spend on things that some might consider a waste of money. We invest in a home, in stocks, in our children's education. We spend money going out to dinner, on a new BMW, on taking vacations. Do you see the difference? Investments appreciate, expenditures don't hold their value.

Mindset is a big component of what we're doing here: You're changing your mindset about marketing and what it could become if you work on it.

The fact is that when your marketing becomes an investment you reinvest as much as you can into it, therefore your practice grows at a predictable pace. That creates more value for the practice. Your practice's valuation increases in the eyes of potential buyers — it's like a little mint. You can predictably forecast what billings will be year after year because of your marketing.

If you don't believe what I'm saying, next time you're speaking with a colleague ask them what they're doing about their marketing. Ask them if they like to market their practice or if they do it begrudgingly. Ask them what kind of returns they're getting on every dollar they spend. Finally, ask them, if they had an extra $100k a year to invest in their practice, how would they allocate it?

My guess is they'll tell you they hate spending on marketing because they don't know what kind of return they get on it or they'll tell you they would never spend that extra $100k on marketing. Congratulations. You now have the upper hand. They're thinking the wrong way about all this.

When you execute this correctly, you're going to dominate.

BUYING BEHAVIORS

- Studies have proven people buy based on emotions and justify their purchases with logical reasoning.
- A buyer is a buyer is a buyer is a buyer, everyone buys for the same reasons.
- Absent of any tangible way for a patient to compare two seemingly identical options, they will make their decision based on price.
- When "shopping" patients don't stop after finding what they want, they will continue and compare.
- When "discovering" something, patients drill down and want to learn more about the specific thing they "discovered," even things they will buy.
- It is far easier to attract a patient when you enter the conversation already going on in their head, or better yet create it.
- To differentiate yourself from the other practices and attract more patients use the A.C.E. principle (Authority, Celebrity, Exclusivity).
- Remember the 10/10/80 phenomenon applies to everything, even your patients.
- Spend more time cultivating the 80 percent that has some level of interest in your practice to double or even triple your new patients without spending more on advertising.

3

IT'S A SYSTEM

"There are no secrets to success.
It is the result of preparation,
hard work, and learning from failure."
— Colin Powell

Look, I know you're used to being the smartest person in the room, the most successful, the one who works the hardest … a winner. It probably frustrates you that, in business, none of these things really matter—the market doesn't give a damn about you and what you're used to. It proves it every time you look at your competitors who are seemingly doing better than you, even though you know you have better outcomes.

Maybe you hear about the new vacation home another practitioner just bought, or the new toy that's in his garage, or about the new building his practice just purchased and moved into. How can they be doing better than you if they're nowhere near as good and don't work as hard?

As I alluded to, the market is a fickle mistress. Relying exclusively on what has gotten you to this point won't get you much further, not unless you don't mind never seeing your family again because you continue to work 12 to 14 hour days. What's going to happen if you continue to do that? You're going to burn out, lose your drive, and wind up hating the one thing that defines who you are and that has brought you so much joy.

Fortunately, this book is showing you that there is an alternative to the way you're doing things. There is a way to create marketing protocols for your practice that generate positive, predictable outcomes each and every time.

This is the chapter where the rubber meets the road. I'm purposely going to paint as stark a picture as possible in this chapter to weed out the docs who just don't "get it." It's kind of like when you sit down with a patient right before a procedure and ever-so-tactfully tell them anything and everything that could go wrong. Well this is it.

I'm going to reset your expectations about what it takes to move your practice to the elite levels. Ready?

A COMPLETE MAKEOVER

What I'm preaching is overhauling your entire marketing program and, instead, creating marketing protocols that need to be executed step-by-step with surgical-like precision (excuse the pun).

I'm not talking about "one and done," these are systematic, sequential campaigns aimed at only your ideal patient. No more "spray and pray." By the time you're done with this chapter, one of two things is going to happen: Either you're going to march into your practice and hand this book to your marketing director because you know they'll get on board with what you're going to do, or you're going to march into your practice and fire your marketing director because you know they won't be on board and you're going to take this on yourself.

Do it yourself? Yeah right! You barely have time now, right? Well, think about it this way, a small investment in your practice now will generate results for years to come. The hidden benefit of doing all this is that once the protocols are in place and working, you'll have more time to handle the marketing because you'll be seeing fewer patients and generating higher revenues because you're attracting more of your ideal patients.

In the long run, systematizing now and creating marketing protocols will afford you more of the liberty that's currently missing from your life. You will be able to cut back the number of hours per day you work and even the number of days a month. You'll be able to do this because, by the time a prospect walks into your practice, you will have already established your A.C.E. and patients will be more than willing to accept a treatment plan as presented regardless of the fee or your competition.

Now don't get me wrong. Up until that point, this system will require that you invest some serious time in thinking through your entire marketing plan for your practice.

Things to consider at this point include:

- Who is my ideal patient? This is key; You must create an avatar, or profile, of who they are.
- What will my message be? Think: Transformation.
- How will I put my message out there? Fish were the fish are; your avatar will help you determine this.
- What will my primary offer be? Again what will resonate with your avatar?
- What will my secondary lead generation offer be? In other words, what kind of lead magnet are you going to create to attract people to your practice? What information are you going to give them for free? This is not about a free consultation, you need something that's very low commitment.
- How will I follow up with leads that request my lead magnet? Will you do this via phone, email, regular mail? The more varied you can be, the better. People respond differently to different media.
- How long will I keep leads active? A good rule of thumb is at least 12 months.
- What will my last-ditch effort be to convert these leads into prospects and patients? This is where you might consider a deep discount before moving leads into quarterly follow ups.

Even if you don't have all the answers to these questions, you'll still be light years ahead of all your competition. You will begin to shift your practice into a systematized positive-outcome, protocol-driven marketing machine.

It's worth mentioning at this point that one of the many benefits of marketing protocols—apart from having more free time—is that you're turning a traditional business expense into a huge moneymaking asset. The more of these protocols that you have in place, the more the value of your practice will increase.

If you can accurately point to any time of year and rattle off what marketing campaign you're running, and what the expected ROI is, your practice becomes more stable. With stability comes a higher return on your life's work should you decide to sell.

But what if you don't want to sell? What if you want to continue to draw an income from the practice into retirement and have it join your portfolio of investments? This can be accomplished as well. What better way to do so than by knowing that you don't need to be in the practice day in and day out because you've taken all the guesswork out of the crucial marketing component?

You see, a practice shouldn't depend exclusively on any one person inside. Yes, you want to have surgeons and staff that are highly skilled and outstanding at what they do. If your practice requires you to be there day in and day out, then all you really have is a very high-paying job — a job with all the traditional constraints and limitations (limited vacation days, restricted income, and the most dysfunctional boss you've ever worked for … you!). Probably not the reasons you decided to strike out on your own right?

Instead, having your marketing under control will allow you to confidently cruise into early retirement, if you like, or to pursue your life's other passions. You'll be confident in your practice's ability to lock out your competition from the minds of your ideal patients because the protocols have proven to do that in the past. You're doing something your competitors can't even begin to wrap their heads around much less attempt.

WHERE TO START?

So there you have it. It's going to be a lot of work and a lot of time invested in creating marketing protocols that competition-proof your business.

For the sake of argument, let's say you're very committed to what I have been saying, but you have no idea where to start. Don't worry, I was in your shoes at one point. I had to learn to generate predictable revenue for my business.

The thing I did that generated the biggest return on my investment was seek outside help and coaching initially. It allowed me to leapfrog years of frustrating trial and error and prevented me from wasting tons of money. Was it expensive? Yes, but the return has exceeded the initial investment many times over.

Seeking outside help allowed me to focus on the operations side of my stores while I "sharpened" my marketing axe, if you will. The coach I brought in to help me became my trusted partner in my journey. Even before I found him, I made a couple of bad decisions when choosing one that I had to quickly terminate, that cost me money and, more importantly, time, but it helped me realize what I did and didn't want in a trusted partner. I will share with you a list that I put together after these trials and errors that will also help you find the right outside partners.

Finally, don't be afraid to ask for help. As a business owner we feel that we have to have all the answers. I can only imagine that it gets amplified when you're a highly skilled surgeon that actually does need to have all the answers. This is simply not true. You will find that, much like in medical school, you need to find a great support system to get you through the difficult times; sometimes it's okay to say you're overwhelmed, sometimes another set of eyes is the best problem-solving tool.

That was the biggest challenge I faced, admitting to myself and the world that I didn't have all the answers and that I was just as clueless at times as anybody else. Luckily, I found the right partner to guide me through the bad times and I came out the other end a much stronger and wiser business owner and businessperson.

THINGS TO CONSIDER AS YOU BEGIN TO SYSTEMATIZE YOUR PRACTICE
The answers to these eight questions will put you light years ahead of the competition.

1. Who is my ideal patient?
2. What will my message be?
3. How will my message reach them?
4. What primary offer will resonate with them?
5. What will my secondary, low-commitment, lead-generation offer be?
6. How will I follow up with the leads that request my lead magnet?
7. How long will I keep my leads active?
8. What will my last-ditch effort be to convert these leads into prospects then patients?

4

A FEW TIPS AND TRICKS

"The secret of business is to know
something that nobody else knows."
– Aristotle Onassis

Since I went into business, I've used many different marketing tactics and implemented my share of campaigns. The majority of these efforts, quite frankly, were fruitless—or at least they appeared to be since I have no idea what kind of ROI they produced.

More recently I've had a few swings and misses, but for the most part, I've been successful.

Let me be clear about one thing right upfront: No one bats 1,000 percent in marketing, at best you're 500 percent. If anyone tells you they're above that, I would seriously question how they're measuring the returns and I would even suspect they were lying to you.

I'm going to share with you couple of campaigns that I've used—and continue to use—that have helped my business grow. I'm going to include real ROI as of the writing of this book and what the next steps are going to be for those campaigns.

As I've mentioned in previous chapters there is a huge gap in the way other marketers tell you how you should market your practice and what I consider to be the foundation for a successful marketing plan. How is my method different? I'm going to take you offline!

There's too much clutter online, too much noise, too many businesses marketing poorly. I don't want you to be one of them. The mere fact that a lot of online marketing like Facebook, email, and Google Adwords is free or almost free makes people rush in without much thought. The barrier to entry by your competitors in these tactics is extremely low. I'm sure you've fielded a ton of calls from salespeople trying to get you to "optimize" your website, "handle" your social media, even "create" online videos for your YouTube channel. These are all good tools, and I use them all, but I use them in combination with offline.

So to be crystal clear, what exactly do I mean when I say offline? An excellent question.

I'm referring to media like direct mail, newspaper ads, even television or radio; basically anything that doesn't require you to turn on your computer to consume.

My favorite of all these media is direct mail. Why? Well, numerous reasons:

- It can be very targeted and personalized.
- It arrives at a prospect's door in a virtually uncluttered environment.
- It forces prospects to interact with it—even if it's just for a second—and it makes them decide if they want to learn more or not before tossing.
- It's inexpensive (by comparison to free or almost free that is) so my competitors are less likely to use it.
- It just flat out works.

Direct mail has been around since the days of the Civil War. No joke. In those days people would receive catalogs from businesses selling their wares. Go back and check it out, not much has changed. You're going to hear from people that direct mail doesn't work, that it's old fashioned, that no one reads their mail anymore. Not true.

Direct mail doesn't work when it's done wrong; when you use a "spray and pray" tactic. True, it's old fashioned, but have you noticed that what's old is constantly new? "No one reads their mail anymore"—this is the biggest myth online marketers want you to believe. What is the first thing either you or your spouse do when you arrive home? You check the mail! Then, if anything catches your attention, you open it immediately. If not, you set it all aside into a pile that you look at later.

Here's the kicker: Every year, thanks to online marketers' practices, mailbox clutter is reduced significantly. That makes the job of cutting through mailbox clutter easier.

Anyway, as you can tell, I'm passionate about direct mail and I encourage all the businesses I work with to espouse it as a very reliable tool for lead generation and repeat sales.

TRIED AND TRUE NEWSLETTERS

So the first example I'm going to share with you is one that, as of this writing, is returning close to $30 in hard sales for every $1 that I spend on it. It's been around for ages, and you've probably seen it done poorly in your mailbox.

As a matter of fact, your relatives or maybe even a member of your family does a much better job of putting one together.

I'm talking about the good old-fashioned newsletter. Our simple, four-page, full color, nothing-fancy newsletter is bringing in close to $30 in documented sales to my businesses. Hard to imagine, right?

You're probably thinking, "Awesome, I'll do an e-newsletter." Wrong! Again, inboxes are getting more and more cluttered. Unless you're putting out a paid, subscription-based e-newsletter to your customers or prospects, chances are if they're pressed for time they're not going to read it. (Think: Delete button.)

On the other hand a physical newsletter must be dealt with and a decision must be made about it. Read and keep, read and toss, or just toss?

We actually put out two different types of newsletters, and if you want to do a newsletter correctly, you should do two as well. But let's start with baby steps.

The first newsletter we issued was to our "house list" of existing customers. The newsletter is not going to win any awards, trust me. It follows the 80-20 rule: it's 80 percent entertaining and informative and 20 percent sales. This is where most of the newsletters you might've gotten in your mailbox get it wrong and where the year-end family newsletters get it right.

The people that do it wrong fill up their newsletters with nothing but industry information and sales pitches and textbook uptight writing. *They teach 100 percent of the time.*

Family newsletters on the other hand are fun and informative, even whimsical—they entertain. The impact of this dichotomy can be illustrated by answering the following question. Who makes more money, a teacher or an entertainer? When your free newsletter is nothing but 100 percent education, readers are going to reach a point where they just don't care about why your new laser is awesome or why the active agent in your chemical peels is new and improved.

Your newsletter needs to entertain first, educate second, and "pitch" last. This is key.

So what should you put in your newsletter to have the success we've had? Here's what's in ours, which you can use as a blue print. There are really only four or five components and they include:

- A piece written by me that talks about what I'm doing in my personal life and sprinkles in marketing advice. I typically find a way to spin what I'm talking about going on in my life into some sort of business/marketing lesson. The pitch varies from very subtle to blatant from time to time. This typically goes on the front page and continues on the inside, forcing your readers to turn the page.
- A feature of a small business or non-profit that does business with us in a question and answer (Q&A) article. This creates all of the content for an entire inside page.
- A silly piece on the life of my many family pets. This can be any sort of entertaining piece. I've seen Sudoku and crossword puzzles used along with funny Internet photos on one of the half of the inside pages.
- A column on the inside of one page containing "odds & ends," which is basically just random information I find interesting and want to share.
- A back page with a "stupid criminals" piece that people love, along with a grilling recipe (did you know that recipe books are the #1 type of book sold?).
- A quick table of contents on the front cover.

So all in all, it's pretty basic.

Don't know what to write? Write about anything that's going on in your life; you don't have to get super intimate. What you'll discover is that the majority of us lead pretty ordinary lives that are basically the same day to day. If you can write about anything outside of what I'm used to doing every day, I'll find it pretty interesting. That may explain the popularity of reality TV shows; we all think that other peoples' lives are much more exciting and interesting than our own.

What you should definitely do with your newsletter is have way to track leads and sales it generates. We use a tracking phone number on them so we can track response rates. That's an example of how, even when you've been at this game as long as I have and have a winning tactic in your toolbox, you can still sharpen that ax to make it better.

Expect to spend about eight to 12 hours the first time you set up your house-list newsletter. This is by far the most time you will invest in it. Every month it should take you one or two hours to generate the content.

A little trick I do is speak into my phone's audio-record feature throughout the month whenever inspiration strikes. When I'm ready to publish, I just email the audio files to my assistant and have her transcribe them. She then emails it back to me and I put on the finishing touches. Takes me about 15 minutes.

To get a sample of the newsletter I use that's bringing close to $30 for every $1 we spend on it, have your office manager **fax "newsletter sample" on practice letterhead to 1-888-316-5887** and I'll be happy to get my template out to you. You can also **request it at my website, www.mgmca.com/newslettersample**, and I'll send one via email.

As I mentioned at the beginning of this section, you really should have two different newsletters. One for your existing clients, which I just went over, and one for all your prospects and unconverted leads. Why do you need to do this? Well, because it gives you an excuse to keep communicating with them.

The way to manage this second newsletter is to create 12, one for every month of the year. These are "canned" newsletters that you can work on once and use forever. Drop prospects and uncovered leads into this mailing list for the next 12 months with the goal of being there once they are ready to schedule a procedure. The main reason people don't buy immediately after meeting with you is not that they're not interested, it's that they may not be ready at that exact moment. You need to make sure you stay in touch with them so that when they are ready you'll be the one they turn to.

After you put someone through the 12-month newsletter sequence, if they still don't schedule a procedure, you can take them off of the list and move them to a less-regular form of follow up.

So what should you include in the 12-month newsletters and how long should they be? For starters, they need to be specific to the time of the year, but not filled with current events so that you can't use them year in and year out.

For a leads newsletter, I recommend a two-page (front and back) newsletter in color. On the front, at the top, should be a small article about what's going on in your office or life that time of year. Again, don't get too "current event," but this could be a perfect article where you further educate your prospect. For example, in January you can write a short "winter healing" piece about healing from a procedure during the winter months in preparation for the upcoming swimsuit season. This creates an open loop, or a way to interest the recipient in reader another issue. You then close this open loop with an "ideal swimsuit styles for different body types" piece in the May issue.

The article on the bottom of the front page of the newsletter should be related to the month itself, like an interesting piece about the origin of Valentine's Day for the February issue or maybe about the origin of Independence Day for the July issue. Again, make this article topical, but not directly drawn from current events.

For the top article on the back side, include a patient success story featuring a transformation of one of your patients. Be sure you get a signed written release from your patient first and let them know how you will be using their story. Split the bottom of the back side of the newsletter into two sections. In one panel, put something fun like Sudoku or a crossword puzzle, and on the other side always put some sort of offer to entice the recipient to return. This offer section might be the only piece that needs to get updated yearly or whenever you change fees, otherwise you can leave the newsletter untouched if you always run the same promotion schedule throughout the year.

Putting these newsletters together shouldn't take more than one or two days. The newsletter can be laid out in a simple program like Microsoft Word, or with the help of a graphic designer if you really want them to have a high-end look.

Remember: You're not trying to win any awards, and the newsletters don't have to be perfect. Their purpose is to keep you in front of your unconverted prospects.

To get a sample of the newsletter I use that's bringing close to $30 for every $1 we spend on it, have your office manager **fax "newsletter sample" on practice letterhead to 1-888-316-5887** and I'll be happy to get my template out to you. You can also **request it at my website, www.mgmca.com/newslettersample**, and I'll send one via email.

If creating your own newsletters proves to be too much of a time investment, you can also work with an outside printer, graphic designer, or marketer. If you do this, make sure that they:

1. Have prior newsletter experience, for themselves and others;
2. Are not just an order taker and that they consult on what would work best;
3. That they will work with you to ensure that the newsletters are written in your voice; they should have a protocol for collecting the content you want to speak about every month and they should make it sound like you actually wrote it;
4. That they can fulfill it for you (mail it) and have a flexible minimum — look for a one-stop-shop so that you don't have to work with one person on the design, another to print the pieces, and a third to mail them.

A small monthly investment will reap huge rewards for your bottom line.

This is the #1 strategy that I force all my clients to adopt because I feel so strongly about it — because I know it works.

Lastly, make sure you publish your newsletter *every month* — not every other month or quarterly. You want it to be such a regular occurrence that when you're late delivering it you have existing clients and prospects calling you up wanting to know why they haven't received their newsletter yet. I'm not joking about this, it actually happens!

INVITATION FOR REPEAT BUSINESS

A second strategy that we've had great success with — and that you can implement immediately at a very low cost — has to do with your past patients. How often do you invite past patients that you haven't heard from in a while to return to your practice? If you don't have some sort of lost customer reactivation protocol in place, *you're leaving tons of money on the table*.

Think about it: These patients are not strangers to your practice. They have already proven to you at least once that they trust you. Wouldn't this be a significantly easier and cheaper sale to make? Often, as business owners, we get so bogged down with the thought of needing new customers that we overlook what's right under our nose. Many of us go so far as to take them for granted, or consider them less valuable.

Well, there are a lot of potential sales to be made by tapping into your existing dormant or lost-customer list. Many of us completely forget about one-and-done customers or customers that stop coming back.

Let me share some interesting statistics about your lost or dormant patients. According to *Medical Practice Insider* over the life of your practice:

- 1 percent of patients will be lost due to death. This is unavoidable there's nothing you can do to prevent it.
- 3 percent of you patients will move away, whether it's to the other side of town or the other side of the world. Unless you have a very compelling reason and a very well-developed relationship with them, chances are you're never going to see them again.
- 5 percent will take a friend's or relative's advice and follow them to *their* preferred practice. Wouldn't it be ideal if yours was the practice people were following their friends to?
- 9 percent of patients will change practices because of price or a better product or service. If you've done your homework in prequalifying your patients via your marketing, then you shouldn't be worried about this. If you are worried, then you're not properly positioning your practice. You're not educating them before and after they do business with you; they don't naturally see you as the best choice.
- 14 percent will leave because they were dissatisfied in some way with their experience while under your care. It could've been something subtle as never having enough parking when they show up to something major like a botched procedure.
- Nearly 70 percent of patients leave due to perceived indifference by you.

The point is, you need to let your patients know, from the very beginning, what to expect when they are under your care and supervision, but you also need to ask them when all is said and done if you met their expectations. Many times this is going to give you feedback on things that you never thought would be deal breakers, but if one person mentions a problem or concern to you, it means that at least 10 other patients had the same concern but they were just too polite to say anything to you.

The feedback patients provide you is gold and negative feedback should be welcomed, not swept under the rug, because it allows you to fix shortcomings that a customer perceives and will make your practice even stronger.

One note here: You're not going to please everyone 100 percent of the time, it's just a fact of life. You can certainly give it your best shot though. Many relationships will be saved just because a patient feels like you care about them being 100 percent satisfied.

The biggest shocker on the previous list is that the majority of you patients, almost 70 percent, leave due to perceived indifference by you. They think you don't care about them.

So how are you showing your patients that you do care? Sometimes all it takes is a little note letting them know you missed them and that you want to invite them back.

This is exactly what we did in my business.

Christmas is the busiest time of the year at my UPS Stores, so one year I decided to invite customers that had shipped with us during the holidays in years past, but didn't return the year prior. The campaign was a winner.

We mailed each of these clients a personalized letter "secretly sent by" my wife. I wrote it in my wife's voice, so it didn't really come from her.

Along with the letter, which was mailed in a plain envelope, we included a "personal check" also "from" my wife. The letter mentioned to recipients that "Victor missed you last year," that she would like to invite them back. Then the letter asked recipients not to tell me about the letter.

The check gave them a dollar discount on purchases over a certain dollar amount.

When the promotion ended, we calculated that the ROI was almost $2 for every $1 we spent. Not setting the world on fire, but to get a promotion right that does more than breakeven is a winner in anyone's book.

We continued to tweak the promotion throughout the year, using it to bring back other lost customers while strengthening the promotion itself. We tested different variables (offer, deadline, even the envelope itself) to try to improve it.

This promotion is now in our regular stable of yearly promotions that perform strongly for us.

If you want to **get a copy of this lost customer campaign**, have your office manager **fax "lost customer sample" on practice letterhead to 1-888-316-5887** and I'll be happy to get it out to you. You can also **request a sample at my website, www.mgmca.com/lostcustomersample** and I'll send you one in the mail so you get the "full" lost-customer experience.

Those are two tactics that I use with existing customers. Now let's look at some strategies I use to attract new customers.

CREATE A FREE BUYING GUIDE

By creating a free buying guide, you make yourself a credible source and the authority in a particular area of your practice.

For example, a buying guide on botox can attract prospective patients who are currently considering injections.

The key is to create a buying guide that contains criteria that only your practice can fully meet. There's a way to do this subtlety without crossing any ethical lines.

For instance, create a list of all your strengths and how you're different from your competition. Then turn each strength and unique item into buying criteria. Let's say, for example, that you have great parking. The way to present this information is to say: "Look for a practice that respects your time and wants to ensure you get in and out of your appointment in a speedy and worry-free manner so you can get on with your busy life."

Remember when I talked to you about features versus benefits? This is exactly what you're doing; you're turning every feature about your practice into a benefit, and then going one step further by turning those features/benefits into content for a buying guide.

Also make sure that you have some features that differentiate your practice from your competitors. For instance, if your practice is the only one that offers guaranteed results on laser tightening with free "touch ups," then mention it, but do it subtlety. For example, say something like, "Reputable practices always offer an extended guarantee on their laser tightening treatments and should provide follow-up to ensure optimum treatment performance."

Now when a prospective patients starts "shopping" for laser tightening treatments, they'll find that your practice is the only one that meets all the criteria.

Using this method of marketing, you've accomplished two important tasks. You've set yourself apart from your competitors by being the only one able to meet all the criteria. More importantly, you've taken the focus off of fee during the shopping process, thus making it harder to compare you to the other practices. Other practices might be cheaper, but they don't meet all the criteria on the buying guide, which in the eyes of the patient makes your practice the most qualified.

The ROI on this tactic is also one of the best for lead generation because of all points I've mentioned: it positions you as the expert, makes you the only logical choice, and makes fee a nonissue when closing a consultation.

WRITE A BOOK

The final tactic that I like to recommend is a little bit more advanced and it definitely is not for the faint of heart, but it will completely blow all your competitors away and can be used for both lead generation and with existing clients. This tactic is writing a book!

Lets' first look at why writing a book is such a great strategy. It all goes back to the A.C.E. principle. It makes you an authority and celebrity that you can convert into exclusivity.

A significant percentage of the American population thinks they can write a book or that they "have a book in them." Thus, our culture—and many others—hold authors in very high regard. People consider authors to be experts in the subject matter that they write about.

Now, when I say the word "book," I don't mean a clinical textbook. I'm talking about a book that is targeted at your prospective patients—not your peers—as a giveaway lead-generation magnet. The focus of the book could be anything you want. For example, maybe you'll decide to discuss case studies from your own experiences that demonstrate how cosmetic surgery changed someone's life for the better. It may take a little research on your part or by someone on your team, but this is time well invested.

Keep in mind while you write your book that, in essence, it's a selling tool. That doesn't mean you should fill it with obvious pitches, but it does need to encourage your prospect to take the next step and come in for an appointment or request further information from your practice.

Writing a book is a stealth way to promote yourself and your practice, and it could even be called the ultimate barrier to entry on your competitor's part.

A hidden benefit of this strategy is that you can launch a public relations campaign based on your book. When you get interviewed, you're pitching your book and not your practice, however, the practice ultimately will get the attention.

The strategy behind marketing protocols for your practice is that you want to take a suspect patient as far away from "shopping" mode as possible. This is why I use the locked room analogy, you let them in and you control what they hear, see, and read. You educate them to shop on something beyond fee to the point that it is nearly irrelevant for your ideal patient.

I think we could all agree that when we're well-informed and highly interested in a product or service we're more price elastic. We make an emotional decision early on in the buying process, and then our mind spends the rest of the time finding rational reasons that justify that decision. A patient's mind goes into justification mode in order to remain congruent with her self-image.

Here's a quick rundown of principles that govern fee elasticity:

- Who is the person or practice doing the selling? How you position yourself and your practice in your market is key because it's all directly related to who you are and *how you're perceived*.
- Who is doing the buying? Different women buy at different price points because of who they are, who they think they are, or who they want to be.
- Where are they buying? This is closely tied to who is buying, meaning a woman who lives in Beverly Hills has a very different, although both affluent, idea of who she is and who she wants versus a woman in Manhattan, New York City.
- How are they buying? The design of the sale's process that leads a woman to your practice *greatly* impacts fee—did you educate them along the way so they see you as a trusted advisor or are you just one of the cheapest games in town? There's a difference, and it matters.

If she is the type of patient that never uses coupons and would never dare, she justifies paying full price for things by telling herself that people in her financial position don't bargain shop. She wants the best and expects to pay for it; she has a sense of pride in who she is.

Affluent patients, which is who you should be targeting by the way, can buy almost anything they want without much thought to price, so to try to lure them with lower fees is counterproductive. Affluent patients are willing to pay top dollar for experiences. Let that sink in … *they are willing to pay more to be an individual who is different from the masses*.

How is your practice positioned to give affluent patients out-of-this-world experiences when they do business with you?

If you start to think of your practice in this manner, you'll be able to position it beyond what your competitors are doing. Everyone has nice facilities and pleasant staff, but what else are you doing to take your patient's experience with your practice beyond the expected? Could you, say, have a luxury chauffeur car service pick her up the day of her procedure? When she wakes up after her procedure, could you transfer her to a 5-star hotel or resort where a personal nurse is at her disposal to ensure all her needs are met those first 24 hours after surgery? Sure, these things cost extra, but they will more than pay for themselves in the form of referrals and return business? Again, don't look at extras like these as expenses, look at them as investments.

An often-overlooked point I would like to make here is that in cosmetic practices the strength of the customer experience hinges on the relationship you have with your staff. Since this isn't a management book, I won't delve too deep on this, but the type of culture you create in you practice *will impact* patient experience.

All the tactics that I mentioned in this chapter serve one purpose and one purpose only: To position you and your practice as the authority in your market, the only logical option a patient would choose when wanting a cosmetic procedure.

We all want to do business with the best possible carpenter, mechanic, landscaper that we can afford; why would it be any different for the medical profession? Building your authority and celebrity will create a larger demand for your practice, at which point you can transition into exclusivity. Then, you can really pick and choose who you work with, when, and at your fee, not the market's.

So to recap: What are you doing in your practice that creates authority, celebrity, and exclusivity?

TOP 4 MARKETING TACTICS
FOR MAXIMUM ROI
And make you an authority and a celebrity to your patients and prospects in the process.

1. Newsletters. One for current patients and one for prospective patients, gets you in front of them and thinking about you when they're ready to schedule.
2. Lost/Dormant Customer Reactivation. They've done business with you once already, why not remind them of that and invite them back? The easiest sale you'll ever make will be the 2nd, then the 3rd, then the 4th, etc.
3. Buying Guide. This will make you an authority on the topic and give you an ethical, but unfair advantage over your competition because you'll be stacking the odds in your favor.
4. Book. The ultimate authority and celebrity creator, guaranteed to give you a prolonged barrier to entry from your competition.

5

HOW TO SELL
WITHOUT SELLING

"The aim of marketing is to make selling unnecessary."
— Peter Drucker

Now let's talk about something that's going to fly in the face of anything you may have been told about selling to date. It may make you a little uncomfortable, but the purpose of this book is put you outside your comfort zone so you can make more money.

Following the masses is rarely the right thing to do if you want to stand out from the crowd. Doing anything in marketing because "everyone does it that way" is a poor excuse for spending money. When you follow industry norms, the only thing you can expect from them are normal results. In order to do things big you have to do things differently. Everything you believe can't be done because "your business is different" can be done if you do things differently.

YOU CLOSE THE SALE

I instruct physician clients to be the ones who close all sales at the end of an initial consultation. Why are you leaving this to your practice manager, treatment coordinator, or maybe another member of your team? Is it because it's "unprofessional" and "no good physician would stoop to this?" Or is it because other consultants have told you that you shouldn't be the one doing it?

The funny thing is that those same consultants don't even take their own advice. They always close their own consultations, they don't trust anyone else to do it for them.

Maybe you hate selling and you hate salespeople. I get it—you didn't spend all those years learning advanced medicine to become a salesman. To put the financial future of you practice in the hands of someone else is just plain missing the point though. I'm sure the person who handles selling to patients at your practice is very skilled and knowledgeable, but unless they're a partner in the practice they have no real skin in the game.

Again, you really are the best person in your practice to close all consultations. Let me tell you why.

For starters, you have the intimate knowledge of the treatment plan you're recommending. Who else but you can answer any possible question a patient could ask about the procedure? You can gauge the situation and put the patient's mind at ease by reassuring her you've done this dozens of times and that she has nothing to be worried about. The other option is your treatment coordinator saying something like: "Gee, I don't know, that's a really good question, I don't think we've ever been asked that. Let me ask the doctor later today and I'll call you and let you know." Would that immediately put your mind at ease as you're about to make to a life-changing decision?

Delaying an answer also doesn't put the practice in a good position. It creates doubt in the patient's mind, they begin to question your abilities, and consider exploring other options.

It also opens the door to trouble later on. If anything goes wrong during or even months after the procedure, through no fault of your own, she's still going to have an opening to blame your practice because her doubt made her question your abilities in the first place.

Another reason for you to do the close is that, when you're the one making the close, it allows you to better diagnose the patient and not over-treat.

For example, maybe during the examination all signs pointed to the patient being a fantastic candidate for liposuction surgery. However, once you've brought her into your office to present the treatment plan you discovered that this patient is better suited for body contouring. Maybe you discover that her emotional state at this moment is not right for the originally recommended procedure. Maybe you discover she's had some adverse reactions during past non-elective procedures that raise a red flag.

Just because the "formal" diagnosis has ended doesn't mean that you should just hand the patient off to someone else to be processed.

A final reason to do your own consultation closings is that potential patients will care more about your practice once they see how much you care. Being present in the room demonstrates to the patient that you empathize with the decision she's about to make and allows you to soothe any anxiety she might be feeling. It lets her see she's not just one in a long line of patients you're treating that day.

Think about your best, high-ticket buying experiences for a minute. The most memorable are the ones where one person walked you through the entire process and answered all your questions. Maybe you even remember the salesperson, or still maintain contact with him?

Remember that affluent patients can buy anything from anyone, but they'll pay top dollar for experiences and for services that make them feel unique. I know you probably would rather hand this portion of the consultation off to someone who's "good at sales." Well this is the wrong way to look at it—you don't acquire a patient to make a sale, you make a sale to acquire a patient. This is just the beginning of your long journey together and any misstep at this early stage could bring it to a screeching halt before it even starts.

Do yourself a favor and close all consultations yourself.

CREATE A CLOSING PROTOCOL

Alright, let's say you absolutely abhor the idea of closing your own consultations. The mere thought sends you into a cold sweat—what should you do? Create a closing protocol so it seems less like selling and more like a procedure you would typically follow. Creating a closing protocol for your treatment plan presentations will help maximize case acceptance. *Don't just wing it.*

First of all, don't call these treatment plans or case presentations in front of your prospective patients—that name sounds sterile and uncaring. I'm sure you can think of a few more suitable names, for example:

- rejuvenation treatment,
- transformation program,
- fountain of youth roadmap.

You get the idea.

This protocol will be developed consisting of three key areas.

First, get a patient to verbalize her burning motivation for wanting this procedure. This may have already been done during the consultation, but get her to verbalize it again. You're doing this so that you can repeat it back to her when you present the treatment plan fee.

Here's a quick example: "We've gone over all the pertinent information regarding the treatment plan, and I believe I've answered all your questions satisfactorily. Are you ready to move forward or is there any other information you need at this time? If you're ready the total investment required to undergo your transformation is $2,000. A small amount to invest for a lifetime of [insert burning motivation here], wouldn't you agree?"

It's that easy, and non-manipulative.

The pitch has a lot of psychological elements in it and even compensates for Thinking or Feeling Myers-Briggs personalities.

By presenting the pitch in this manner, the patient is being reminded why she wanted to undergo this transformation using her own words.

Next, you need to future pace your patient to what life will be like after the procedure and after the recuperation process. You can do this via videos, photos, or written testimonials.

At this point, your focus should be on selling the transformation. Have the patient envision her life one year from now. It sounds hokey, but you might even want her to close her eyes to create a clear mental picture. Then have her repeat back to you what she saw in as much detail as possible.

This plays well with the first point I made about her burning motivation. When you attempt to close a patient, if you can have her visualize her life with the product, then subconsciously she has already bought it.

Why do you think auto dealerships take you out for a test drive? So you can visualize your life with the car. How it feels. How awesome you look in it. All the heads you're turning.

Future pacing will do this for your patients, it's your practice's equivalent of going for a test drive.

Lastly, you need to have thought through all the objections ahead of time and have come up with a way of eliminating them. There are different ways to do this.

The one I use and that's worked like a charm for me is to use simple 3-by-5-inch index cards. As you're developing your closing protocol, list all the objections you can possibly think of on 3-by-5-inch index cards and put them on a table in front of you. On the back of the cards, list keywords you will use to overcome each objection.

Let me give you an example, one that I know you face often.

"The fee is much more than I was prepared to spend." If you did your pre-selling correctly, this shouldn't be an objection you hear a lot at close time. If you are hearing it consistently, you need to go back and sharpen your pre-consultation selling ax. Occasionally this objection does sneak through—even the most affluent people at times take pride in finding what they perceive to be "the best deal in town."

One way to overcome this objection is by offering Care Credit for 100 percent or a portion of the fee. Another way would be to break the billing up into two or three payments. Still another is to have a down sell, where the patient gets something like what she came in for but not with all the bells and whistles (i.e. lipo vs. body sculpting). Maybe offer an alternative treatment plan that only has one procedure instead of two or three.

Whatever you do, don't get defensive and start trying to justify your fee. At that point, you're a used car dealer haggling with someone on the lot. You're not a used car dealer right?

Your fees are well earned and, if you do amazing work, you should charge top dollar for it. Never bargain!

EVERYTHING SPEAKS

As you prepare you closing protocol one often overlooked piece of this very important puzzle is staging. Where do you close a patient?

A lot of practices don't give this any thought, but some of the best usually use a "closing room."

A "closing room" is nothing more than an office at your practice that is used for nothing but closing. You don't take private phone calls there, your kids and spouse don't use it to hang out when they're waiting for you at the office, and you certainly don't use it day in and day out.

It's a stage where you deliver some of the most important performances of your career.

So what should you have in this "closing room" and what do you do once you're in it to get a positive outcome?

Well, the room should ideally look like an office that you would use except without the clutter. On the walls you want to have three—and only three—strategically selected and placed pieces that your patient can admire when you step out of the room because you "accidentally" left something in the exam room.

Why three, you ask? A mind that's given too many pieces of information at one time is overloaded and shuts down, and a confused mind will always say "no."

On the walls I recommend placing a photo of your family with a dog, if you don't have a dog borrow one for the photo, this will make you come across as trustworthy and likeable.

Also place your degree on the wall—if you went to a prestigious university or medical school—along with any other distinction you've been awarded. Did you get a personal letter from the President thanking you for all the awesome pro-bono work you do? Post it! This is right up A.C.E.'s alley.

Lastly, post the most dramatic, gut-wrenching, heartfelt testimonial letter you've ever received. It doesn't matter if it's older, what you want is something that really tells the story of how you changed someone's life for the better. This acts as social proof to your patient that they made the right decision by working with you.

When you're with your patient, don't sit behind the desk. Start off the consultation behind the desk but quickly move to a position beside your patient. The key here is that you want nothing in between you and your patient's heart lines.

This will again make you come across as warm and trustworthy because you're now seen as someone who is working *alongside* the patient instead of in *opposition* to her (as you are when you're sitting across from her).

Now you're ready to proceed with your close.

KEEP THE MOMENTUM

So you've answered all the questions, handled all the objections, and you still have no commitment from the patient. Now what?

In my experience, one of two things will keep the sale moving forward.

First, ask the patient if she has any other questions or concerns that she might not have expressed. If she mentions anything, you should always answer: "That's a great question. Now let me ask you one before I answer it. Is this there any other question you have that you might be reluctant to ask right now? Don't worry, there is no such thing as a dumb question, so please feel free to ask me anything."

Objections are just unanswered questions; you might have to dig a little deeper and to get to the root of the question or objection.

The second and the most prevalent thing that might keep a sale from happening after all initial objections have been handled is money.

If a patient expresses to you that she has no other questions and you feel that you've made the patient feel at ease but she is still reluctant to move forward, it might be that she is afraid to say that she can't afford the procedure.

At this point, you need to use great tact in offering an alternate plan that might be more in line with the patient's economic expectations. Without uttering phrases like "Is the fee to much for you?" or "Is this more expensive that what you had thought it would be?," carefully steer the patient toward a down sell to save the sale and not be perceived as arrogant by taking a "take it or leave it" like stance.

Whatever happens, by all means — as I've covered before — do not sit there and start discounting. If your patient lead-generation process has been designed right, then you should have very few of these types of prospective patients come through your doors.

Once you've developed a protocol for closing that takes into consideration the elements I just mentioned, you can wash your hands of the whole process right?

Wrong. The most important part of this protocol is implementation and testing.

Let's be realistic: Your whole career is based on protocols and their successful implementation. How do you implement and test those?

Here's what I recommend my clients do in their closing consultations if they absolutely must delegate this down the road.

Sit in while your treatment coordinator delivers them at the beginning then do "spot checks" at different intervals throughout the month. Look ... people respect what you inspect. If it looks like you don't care about the protocols you worked hard to create, then your staff may not either.

Sit in during the presentations and objectively analyze your patient's reaction to different components of the close. This way you can refine any aspect where there appears to be resistance, further develop your staff on how to appropriately answer questions that may come up, or even just test the sequence in which you present your treatment plan.

The big takeaway is that, once you have your protocol and it appears to be working well, you can start to test different components of it to optimize it. When I say optimize, I mean the ROI it generates, not necessarily the number of procedures you schedule from it. Make sure you only test one component of the closing protocol at a time so you can get a clear understanding of the impact of the tested component. Your testing period should be two to four weeks to give you enough of a sample size, unless you have a large-volume practice, in which case, one to weeks should suffice.

In summary, I can't stress this enough: The selling process for your practice begins the minute a suspect patient interacts with your marketing campaign for the first time. If you wait until you get the patient into your office, you've done yourself a huge disservice and will spend the entire consultation swimming upstream because every step of the way, the patient will have price on her mind and will focus on little else.

When you realize that selling begins from the first second, you're doing yourself and your practice a huge favor. Firstly, you'll be able to sell without selling to your prospective patients. Secondly, you'll exude confidence when you start talking fees with your patients. You'll sell without coming across as pushy or desperate because at every step of the education of your prospect you've held her hand as you positioned yourself to be the authority in your field. You've taught her that selecting a surgeon based entirely on fee is penny wise and dollar foolish.

Since you're charging premium fees and have established yourself as the local authority, you become a celebrity in her eyes. As such, you must practice exclusivity, demonstrating that you are going to only work with patients that are just as motived as you are to have the best possible outcome from their transformation. This allows you to charge more because you're very selective about who you "partner" with.

In short, what you are trying to accomplish is to elevate your practice above your competition, which is likely disorganized and leaves the treatment plan presentation to chance or just "wing it."

You already have protocols for all the procedures your preform, consider your marketing as just another procedure in your practice and develop a protocol that you never deviate from. If you do nothing else I suggest in this book, this one thing will more than double your practice's income over its lifetime.

Don't forget: People respect what you inspect. If you're not closing consultations yourself, be sure to inspect results to make sure protocols are being followed.

TIPS TO CLOSING THE CONSULTATION

1. If you don't want to feel like you're selling because it makes you nervous, create a closing protocol and view it as just another procedure that you follow.
2. Staging is key and so are the surroundings; everything speaks. If you don't have a "closing room," get one ASAP.
3. Future pace your patients and have them tell you how their life will be different one year after the procedure so they commit mentally.
4. The heart line is of utmost importance. Be sure nothing is in between you and your patient. Come out from behind the desk and sit near or next to her.
5. Have your patient tell you when you step into your closing room why she wants this procedure. This answer is something you can remind the patient of when you present your fee.
6. Objections are just unanswered questions. Use 3-by-5-inch index cards with all possible objections and come up with a game plan for handling them.
7. If a patient can't enunciate to you why she's not ready to move forward, it's probably about the fee. Down sell or offer options, don't negotiate or discount.
8. If you absolutely must delegate closing after creating your closing protocol, always inspect—people respect what you inspect.

6

A CULTURAL TRANSFORMATION

"If you don't drive your business,
you will be driven out of business."
— B. C. Forbes

Be the practice and the practice will become you! What does this mean?

What I'm talking about here is for you to become the face of your practice.

I have first-hand experience with this; I became the face of all of my UPS Stores.

I mean, who wants to do business with a brown three-letter symbol? No one! They want to buy their cuts of beef from Alex the butcher, have Sabrina the stylist help them pick out their next suit, and they definitely want to know that Carol their general practitioner is keeping them healthy.

In order for me to transform my business, my family and I had to become its face.

There are several ways that I accomplished this, which I won't really delve into (although the aforementioned newsletters was one of them).

What I discovered as a result of making this transformation was that people started calling my stores to personally ask for me because the wanted to tell me how much they enjoy me marketing to them.

Let me say that one more time: They call my stores to thank me for sending them advertising! Yeah, chew on that for a while.

As a matter of fact I just had a call today with a customer complimenting me on a recent promotion I did. I was only able to accomplish this because I gave my customers a face and a real family that they can connect with my business. They know that, behind the UPS logo, there is a real person that truly cares about them and that lives in their community.

Maybe you're thinking: "That's great for you, but I'm a surgeon. That's not what we do."

All the more reason for you to do it. If all of your competitors are hiding behind a glossy, polished, professional image, think of the breath of fresh air that you would be by presenting yourself as a regular person, someone who buys groceries where your patients buy groceries, has children in the same schools, gasses up at the corner station, and worries about the same things as they do. That kind of image will make you, the physician, and by default your practice, more approachable and relatable.

If you're afraid that people won't be interested in you then you'll be pleasantly surprised to know that a lot people consider their lives "ordinary" and "unexciting." As I speculated before, this may be the main reason why reality TV is so prominent today; people want to live vicariously through the experiences of others. An event in your life or practice that might seem commonplace to you might be big news to someone who hasn't seen it a hundred times before.

The fact is, we all want to do business with people we know, like, and trust. Who is the person that we all know, like, and trust the most? Ourselves! If you present yourself to your prospective patients as being just like them, they are more likely to do business with you because they feel they can relate to you on some level.

If the end you foresee for your career involves selling your practice, then over time, you will want to fade slowly into the background as the face of the practice and make the practice itself the celebrity. The other members of your staff can still be featured in its promotions, but overall you want the practice itself to be known as the place to go for cosmetic procedures. You accomplish this by continually improving the expertise of the practice itself and its people.

This might sound contradictory to what I stated earlier about becoming the face of your practice, but this is a winning strategy to follow. The reason you want to fade into the background and allow the practice to become the celebrity is that, in time, you won't want its financial future tied directly to you or any other physician on the staff. Instead, you want to create a reputation of always hiring the best and most experienced surgeons money can buy, and that being treated by any of them is being treated by the best. Of course, you have to make sure you can deliver on this philosophy, but I'm sure that through careful staff selection and development this can be achieved.

WORTH THE EFFORT

At the end of the day, putting the strategies I shared with you into practice is a lot of work and commitment. But trust me, once you have them in place and start seeing positive outcomes from them, you'll realize that the time you've invested has been well worth it.

The value of these strategies will be compounded over the years as you find that you can dust off winning protocols that you hadn't used in a while, update them, and get good results just as you were getting before.

What you're creating is evergreen assets for your business. While I've labeled them "tactics" and "protocols" and "strategies," what they ultimately are is assets when it comes time to sell your business.

Imagine preparing to sell your practice as you wind down your career and having a host of prospective buyers interested in your practice because it's the most successful in town. Your price is premium, but fair, because it accurately reflects the lifetime of investments you've made in it. You sit down with potential buyers share with them your money-making protocols, all which back up your asking price and project a very healthy, constant, continued growth for the years to come.

At that time, you could have the pick of the litter, so to speak, among the buyers; in essence they would need to justify to you why you should sell to them instead of the other way around. If you choose not to sell your practice, but to instead keep it as a continuous source of income without having to be involved in the day to day, then these protocols will also help you accomplish that goal.

These protocols will competition-proof your practice because you will be able to attract only your ideal patients like bees to honey. You will know exactly what kind of revenue you can expect from your marketing protocols, month in and month out, making it easier to attract top talent to keep your practice going while you enjoy your life.

Even if you decide to close the practice down at the end of your career, these protocols will make it easier to start prepping for that a few years in advance. You'll be able to adjust the dial on your marketing protocols to better match the hours that you want to work and the number of patients that you want to see. You'll remove the feast-or-famine of having to take every patient because no one else might show up. You can become very selective and truly exclusive in who you let in your doors. A *hidden benefit* of this is that you can continue to raise your fees as you taper off the number of patients you see, so you'll avoid any real drop in income or lifestyle. In short, you'll be able to work less and make the same amount of money as before.

What I'm laying before you may seem like a pipe dream, but it is very possible.

However, it is not without some serious upfront investment of time and resources on your part.

I know you have what it takes to undergo this transformation; if there's one thing you have, it's the commitment and drive to be the best surgeon you can be. Your drive and commitment are what got you through your undergrad years, med school, your internship and residency, and then your fellowship.

Doing what I'm proposing is nowhere near as mentally and physically grueling as all those years were. It does require tapping into the mindset, the hunger, you had during that part of your life. You know it's still in you or else you wouldn't have picked up this book. Am I assuming too much? I don't think so, and I'm willing to bet neither do you.

What you're looking for at this point in your career might be just getting home in time to have dinner with your family an extra night or two every week. You've worked to achieve your current level of success, now I want to make it easier on you to continue building on what you have thus far.

What I'm proposing in this book can remove those "golden handcuffs" you may be finding yourself shackled with and truly give you your life back. You'll get more enjoyment out of what you do, and remember why you went into cosmetic plastic surgery in the first place.

Marketing protocols can help you achieve whatever level of success you desire. All you have to decide on is what you want and how hard you're willing to work to get there.

THE CELEBRITY TREATMENT

If you don't believe that becoming the face of your practice works with your patients let me share a story I call "the birthday party."

A few months ago, I was at one of my stores in Albuquerque, N.M., working the counter for a week. It's something I do to stay in touch with my customers and to have boots on the ground.

While I was there, a mother walked in with a little girl no more than 2 years old who was going through her "no" phase.

I waited on her and as we were talking she mentioned to me that I looked very familiar, but she couldn't remember from where.

As we kept talking she glanced over to my nametag and read my name, that's when it hit her like a ton of bricks.

"Oh my God, *YOU'RE Victor!* You're the guy from the postcards and newsletter! We *love* getting your stuff, *it's so different!*"

I thanked her for recognizing me and thanked her for being a repeat customer, but she wasn't finished telling me how much they enjoyed my advertising. She said, "My daughter," who by this point was back in the car with grandma, "has been walking around the house for the last month with the invitation you sent us to your 'birthday party'."

The month before I ran a "birthday party" store promotion and I sent out realistic "invitations" to my house list.

"She refuses to put it down or let us take it from her," my customer continued. "She says she's going to 'Victor's party'. Wait until I get back to the car and I tell her I just met Victor from the 'birthday party', she's going to love it!"

Again I thanked her and asked her to tell her daughter "hello" for me. By this time I was a little embarrassed, I admit, because of all the attention, but the other customers in the store really liked the story and thought what I was doing was awesome. *Two of them even asked me put them on them on my mailing list,* so that I can *market* to them.

If this story doesn't convince you of the impact these type of marketing protocols can have in differentiating you from your competitors, I'm not sure anything else will.

Incidentally, later that same week I had an older gentleman also recognize me in the store and tell he, "didn't think I was real," but was glad I actually existed and he got to meet me.

Talk about getting the celebrity treatment in Albuquerque that week.

7

HOW TO FIND THE RIGHT MARKETING PARTNER

"Even if the chef has a good business head,
his focus should be behind kitchen doors.
A business partner should take care of
everything in front of the kitchen doors."
– Bobby Flay

I realize that you are probably already under tremendous pressure and time constraints at your practice, so the last thing you're looking for is something else to put on your plate. So let me talk for a minute about ways to avoid the "do-it-yourself" approach, which will result in nothing getting implemented and things staying exactly the same.

First of all, let's analyze your current situation. Here is a checklist that I use with clients to try to and help them find weak spots in their practice that are preventing them from getting the results they're looking for. If you'll indulge me for a minute and go through it I promise it will be worth your while.

How many of these items apply to your practice? <u>Place a check mark next to those that do.</u>

☐ You're actively marketing your practice

☐ You focus your marketing primarily on online advertising

☐ You're involved in the marketing decisions your practice makes.

☐ The person directly responsible for marketing your practice is not a spouse, relative, or friend

☐ The person directly responsible for determining your marketing strategy has prior marketing experience.

☐ You're currently at least asking all new patients how they heard of you

☐ You have a sales protocol for all prospect patients that you meet with to ensure you follow up with all of them and that you maximize your net scheduling rate.

☐ You check your conversion numbers religiously and can tell me with a fair amount of certainty what your ROI is on your different advertising investments.

☐ You are continually looking for weaknesses in your practice so you can address them and make them better.

☐ You have a mentor, coach, mastermind group that you can bounce ideas off of.

If you found that **seven or more** of these items apply to your business, congratulations, you're not too far from achieving the results you want. If you can carve out some time from your schedule, even if it's one hour, two or three days a week, you should be able to create a basic marketing protocol for your practice in about 30 days. I know 30 days sounds like a long time, but the time is going to pass anyway, so why not spend a small portion of it working *on your practice instead of in it?*

If you found that **between five and six** of the questions apply to your practice, then you're are at a critical point in the life of your practice. The decisions you make in the coming six to 12 months will have a ripple effect that will impact the direction your practice continues to develop in.

At this point, what I recommend is that you really sit down and think through a lot of the questions that I asked in the book and why you don't have better answers for them. Do you not have enough time? Do you not know where to start?

Then my suggestion is to bring someone into your practice to help you or your marketing director implement a simple marketing protocol that can take you from lead generation to closing the consultation and referral generation.

There are many well-qualified professionals out there that specialize in working with cosmetic practices. They understand your challenges and know exactly what to do to help make this transition as easy as possible for you. Later on in this chapter I'm going to be sharing with a "buying guide" for hiring your first or your next marketing specialist.

Back to the list above. If you found that **fewer than five** of the questions apply to your practice, I applaud you for still being in business. You, my friend, are a survivor! You're what I like to call a "hustler." The kind of person that never quits, puts his head down, and gets the job done no matter what.

You're also probably the surgeon working 60 to 70 hours per week, never having a minute to even eat lunch, and whose family life is falling apart or nonexistent.

On top of that, your practice is probably barely scraping by.

Don't worry, I was in the same shoes you're in now only a few years ago.

Granted, I wasn't a surgeon, but I was working day and night and on the verge of my second divorce.

AN EVOLUTION

I'm going to take a minute to speak to you the "hustler", grinding to make $100,000 a year, in a no-nonsense way, because sometimes this is exactly what we need to hear. I don't want to offend you, but you need to wake up.

You need to get your head out of your work long enough to look around and realize you need help. And you need to find someone to help you now. And I mean yesterday.

Stubbornly believing that you don't need help is not a strategy for future growth!

I say this with all due respect because this is exactly who I was. I couldn't see the forest for the trees, and thought that if I just worked harder and longer, then things would pan out. Well, they didn't and I almost lost it all. Here's what I did to turn things around:

- I scoured the Web and poured over books and magazines to learn as much as I could about marketing.
- I adopted a realistic view of myself and identified my weaknesses that were keeping me from being successful.
- I invested in myself, something I do 'til this day, because I knew then that it would payoff tenfold.
- I found someone who I could trust to partner with me and help me get me and my business back on track.

Slowly, and with a lot of hard work on my part, I was able to turn my business around.

The only regret I have from doing it the way I did was that I didn't realize then that I was losing so much time by trying to do it all myself.

At the beginning I had no other choice but to implement on my own; I couldn't afford to pay anyone else to do it for me. The coaching and consulting I was getting was already a stretch, and to throw another expense on top of that back then would've been like adding gasoline to a fire. Instead, I had to be resourceful.

Unfortunately, I got so good at being resourceful that when I started making money and being able to afford outside help, I still didn't get it. I didn't think I needed it. Looking back, I realize that if I hadn't had gotten so good at being resourceful and invested a little more in myself and my business, I could've shaved months off the recovery period.

Sounds like a horror story, doesn't it? At the time it was, but it's also an accurate portrayal of who I was back then.

That's what you need to accept in order to save your practice; it's going to take a change of mindset.

The huge difference and the biggest thing in your favor is that your average sale is much larger than mine, so your recovery should be significantly shorter than mine. I had to recover my businesses $50 to $100 at a time; trust me, that was a lot of sales.

I estimate that being resourceful cost me about $10,000 to $20,000 per year, per store. That's not a huge amount individually, but when you own multiple stores it adds up quick.

Marketing is the "heart" of your practice, it's what sustains all the other "organs" and keeps blood pulsing through them. If you fail to take care of your "heart" your practice will one day die.

WHY WORK WITH AN OUTSIDER?

There are a number of reasons why working with someone that is not directly dependent on your practice might be the best course to take.

The *Harvard Business Review* cited the study, "Integrating Problem Solvers from Analogous Markets in New Product Ideation" published by the journal Management Science in late 2013, in which it was revealed that, "it might pay to systematically search across firm-external sources of innovation that were formerly out of scope" and that "searching in far versus near analogous markets" provided better results. Furthermore, the study found that, "it might pay to systematically search across firm-external sources of innovation that were formerly out of scope."

Besides the obvious reason of being able to be more objective—not emotionally attached to any one person or thing—the biggest advantage an independent consultant brings to the table is years of experience earned by trial and error. About 80 percent of my experience was earned working on my own business, the remaining 20 percent is best practices I've picked up along the way while working with clients.

Many times, by working clients outside your own industry, a consultant is able to tap into a greater knowledge and experience base.

In the long run working with a seasoned, outside professional will save you time and money. Just about every professional has one or two quick strategies that they can implement in your practice that will give an immediate result. If you're looking for a place to cut corners and save money, there are better areas to look than marketing.

There is no honor in doing everything in your practice by yourself. Conservatively, your time is worth anywhere from $100-$500 per hour. A good consultant's hourly fee will be about the same, however, his fees can be amortized over many years because the protocols he develops and you implement can remain in place with only minor tweaks being required.

A major benefit that is often overlooked when trying to justify the investment in outside help is that outside help brings you speed of implementation. How many times has this happened: You come up with a great marketing idea over the weekend or late in the day for your practice, saying to yourself you'll work on it tomorrow, but tomorrow never comes? Then, the idea dies before it even had a chance to live. Most of the time it's just because you were too busy and you didn't have time to flesh it out. You walk into your practice on Monday morning, and before you know it you're elbows deep in crocodiles. I get it, I've been there.

With a consultant, you don't have to worry about this. Most consultants can handle all the project details from start to finish after a session with you. Or they work alongside you—if that's your preference—handing you the tools you need as you move along.

Why is speed so important? Because the number one enemy of any great idea is time. The more time that is spent from when the idea came to you, to when you actually implement the idea, the more likely you'll do nothing about it. Running a close second to time is the need to fail fast. You read that right, you want to fail fast. This allows you to make necessary changes to your idea, instead of wasting time and money getting something perfect, only to find out it's a colossal failure. In marketing, you have to be okay with failing fast; just take your lumps, learn your lesson, and correct your course for the second go round.

BUYING GUIDE

So I promised to give you a "buying guide" you can use if and when you decide to bring someone into your practice to help you or completely take over the marketing function and create protocols.

> A printable, digital version of this can be found at
> **www.mgmca.com/guide**

Here are seven key questions every marketing and advertising consultant must be able to answer to create marketing protocols for your practice that will guarantee you get the biggest ROI bang for your buck.

1. **Do you currently have marketing protocols in your business to generate new and repeat business? Tell me about it.**

The answer to this question is key. What you're listening for specifically is whether the consultant has an understanding that marketing is more than just a shotgun, feast-or-famine, slash-and-burn event.

Key words or phrases they might use if they have no marketing protocols in place are:

- Cold-call, network, or canvas
- Social media, Facebook, or Twitter
- I'm out on calls all day.
- What we do is different.
- We work with anyone.

The reason the answer to this question is important is that you can't expect someone, or a company, who has no understanding of how to create effective marketing protocols to help your practice implement effective marketing protocols. Let me put it another way, would you go to a smoker for advice or help to quit smoking?

You want to partner with some who uses protocols to generate a steady stream of new and repeat business. Someone who works to attract only the best customers for their business. Someone who works smarter not harder. In business, unfortunately, effort and hustle is not something you can deposit in the bank, but I know you're painfully aware of this, you've been working hard for years.

A company that is not willing to invest the time and the effort to set itself apart from the herd will have a very hard time doing the same for you. The beauty of complexity is that it gives the owner a built in defense against competitors. People don't want to do what's hard; we all want to do what's easy. You pay for easy in subpar, disappointing results.

2. Have you been trained by a pioneer and an authority in marketing and do you belong to his insider's circle?

Again the answer to this question will give a lot of useful information that will help you make the correct partnership decision. If you got a negative answer to question #1 you almost always also get a negative answer to this question.

What you're looking for here is someone who has learned from the best in the industry. By doing this you leapfrog years of trial and error with the wrong partner and use only strategies and tactics that have been proven to make money.

You want a partner that's going to offer direct, unlimited access to the guru himself by belonging to their inner circle. The ability to speak daily, if necessary, with other professionals in this industry will also let you have access to them. You pay for one and get one hundred!

3. How are you continually expanding your knowledge? And how are you using what you have learned?

This is a tricky one. Any company or professional worth their salt will invest in training. So expect to hear a positive response. You of all people understand the importance of continuing to sharpen your ax as technology continues to evolve.

What you drill them on is how they are using what they're learning to help their clients make money as well. It's a partnership, remember?

This takes a lot of out-of-the-box thinking. Normally, businesspeople look at something and, if it's not directly in their industry, they dismiss it as "won't work for me." What you want to hear is that people are asking themselves "How can I make this work for me?" Then, it's only a short hop to the next logical question, which is "How can I use this with my clients?" You follow what I'm saying here?

A narrow, unimaginative mind always looks for the easiest answer—the path of least resistance. As I mentioned before, easy gives you no defense against competition. The harder something is to duplicate, the more built-in defenses it will have and the longer you will have the edge. Breakthroughs almost always come from outside, from borrowing and adapting.

Always look for a partner that is continually growing, not just to pad their own wallet, but to pad the wallets of their clients. Someone who is spreading the wealth.

4. Do you partner exclusively with one practice per market?

I won't beat around the bush here. It's unethical and a conflict of interest to have more than one horse in your stable. Anyone who argues the opposite is dead wrong.

Remember, this is a partnership. One where both parties get positive outcomes and are loyal to each other. If not, who gets the killer new marketing idea? You can't cut the baby in half.

These days, this practice is the standard in marketing, so I wouldn't expect you to hear a negative answer to this. Unless, of course, the fees they're charging you aren't "substantial enough." What they're saying here is that you're giving them enough money to date you, but not to marry you. Gives new meaning to "can't buy me love," huh?

You want a true partner, someone who is as committed to your success as you are. You want an extension of your practice that will be with you no matter how much you paid them last month. Someone who will be there as long as your relationship is as beneficial for you as it is for them. Then and only then can you really call it a partnership.

Warning: Anyone who starts any type of relationship with a long, undefined contract is probably only looking out for themselves. They are telling you from the very beginning that if things go bad they will collect! Doesn't exactly scream partnership does it?

5. What kind of "done for you" and "done with you" services do you offer?

The answer to this question may seem obvious to both you and any prospective partner you're questioning but, like an onion, it has layers. You expect that the company you choose to partner with does offer "done for you" and "done with you" services.

I mean, they don't expect you to shoot your own commercial or design your own ad or billboard. The thing is, this is not "done for you" or "done with you" service. This is doing what you've paid them to do.

The kind of "done for you" and "done with you" service I'm talking about is capturing all of your leads, prospects, and suspects. Delivering leads is easy. What do you do about the prospects and suspects that don't exactly scream out to you that they're interested?

Remember that at any given time only about 10 percent of your target market is ready to buy immediately. Another 10 percent is not and will never be interested. So what do you do about the other 80 percent that has some level of interest?

This is where the real money is made. Moving these 80 percent from suspects to prospects to leads then finally to patients is what a "done for you" and "done with you" service is all about.

Think about it. You paid to reach 100 percent of your target market. Why are you leaving selling to up to 80 percent of them to chance, hoping that they remember you when they're ready to pull out their wallet? Why are you not nurturing any type of relationship with them?

The right partner understands these facts and will help you capture as much or as little of that remaining 80 percent as you want. Failure to follow up is failing to plan. Failure to plan is planning to fail.

6. Do you offer or coordinate ongoing education or mastermind groups where I or a member of my practice can share ideas with other practices?

I don't expect you to get a positive response to this question. In fact, I expect you to get a blank stare, or maybe some mumbles about that "not really being what we do."

If you do get a positive response, please share it with me. These are the types of companies I want to do business with. A company that will invest in me as much as I am investing in them.

I keep going back to it, but it should be a partnership where both parties grow and learn and benefit. The more educated I am as a consumer about what you do, the better of a customer I will be and the easier I will be to work with.

A true partner should not be afraid to lift the veil and let you peak behind the curtain to show you how they do what they do. On the contrary, a true partner should help you make the connections you need to be more successful. Have I mentioned that almost all business breakthroughs come from outside their industry? There's real power in mastermind groups. Harness it.

7. Do you offer a 100 percent money back results guarantee?

This one is really simple. Can your "partner" put his money where his mouth is? A no-holds-barred, anything-goes, 100 percent refund of each and every single penny paid if they don't deliver the results they promised?

Talk is cheap. A potential partner that is not willing to lay it all out on the line and back his claims is either:

- Not very good at what they do.
- Greedy and hates losing money, which is probably because they're not very good at what they do.
- Is not really interested in forming any sort of long-term partnership with you and your practice.

A printable, digital version of this can be found at
www.mgmca.com/guide

I understand you can't win all the battles, but you must have the confidence that your army will not desert you and retreat at the first sign of defeat. Or that it won't hide behind a contract that you signed while on a "We'll give you the sun and moons" high!

It's not complicated. I made a lot of bad marketing investments before I learned what I was doing. Not once did I get even a, "sorry, better luck next time" phone call, email, or text from any of my "partners." They got paid and I got screwed! Don't let that happen to you!

LET US HELP YOU

Now that you have your buying guide—and most importantly, now that you have a better understanding of the significance of marketing protocols for your practice—I would like to extend you a one-time offer as a show of gratitude for purchasing and reading my book.

I invite you to learn more about how we can help your practice differentiate itself from the others, attract more of your ideal patients, and enjoy a better work-life balance without your practice's bottom-line suffering.

I am offering to work with you and **help you implement your first marketing protocol with no upfront fee**. I'm willing to put my money where my mouth is, and if you don't make any money, I don't make any money.

Why am I doing this? Well because I've found that the majority of physicians, and business owners for that matter, do little or nothing to implement what they've learned after reading a book, attending a seminar, or taking a class. They get a ton of notes and ideas, then life happens when they return to their practice. They get busy, their staff talks them out of it, or they try to find a "better" time to implement. The excuses go on and on. I offer you speed of implementation, and money loves speed.

If you would like **to take me up on this offer please call fax "cosmetics book diagnostic consultation" on your practice letter head to 1-888-316-5887** to schedule a diagnostic call with me so I can learn a little bit more about your practice and your long term goals.

Please be sure to include an email address where we can contact you directly and a best time to call to schedule the appointment.

While scheduling the call we will take a $300 deposit that is 100 percent refundable after we've had the call.

Why the fee? Two reasons: One, my time is valuable and have limited inventory, so I have to place a value on it regardless of what I do; and two, it guarantees that you will show up for the call—this goes back to my limited inventory, I can't resell that hour to someone if I've set it aside for you.

After scheduling the call, you'll receive a short five-question survey so I can learn a little bit more about your practice and determine if you're a good candidate for my help. If we're a fit, then I'll be happy to get to work with you immediately.

If this **sounds like too big of a commitment**, I understand. Remember: Only 10 percent are ready to take you up on any offer right now, that's why **I have something for you as well.**

You can **go to www.mgmca.com/toolkit and download our cosmetic practice makeover toolkit**. In it you will find samples and templates of all the different pieces and strategies I discussed in this book. Many of these are near fill-in-the-blank pieces where, with some minor modifications, you can start using them immediately. They are **100 percent copyright free**.

I only ask two things: that you don't use them exactly as you get them in order to set your practice apart from others who take me up on this offer; and that you **share your results with me by faxing them to 1-888-316-5887 or by emailing them to info@mgmca.com**. That way, I can either make them stronger or, with your permission, I can share your successes with other like-minded physicians that are just starting and need encouragement.

BUYING GUIDE

Use this before making any future purchase or signing any contract with a marketer, consultant, or advertising agency. See pages 68-72 for instructions on using this guide.

Business Name: _____ Date: _____

1. **Do you currently have marketing protocols in your business to generate new and repeat business? Tell me about it.**

2. **Have you been trained by a pioneer and an authority in marketing and do you belong to his insider's circle?**

3. **How are you continually expanding your knowledge? And how are you using what you have learned?**

4. **Do you partner exclusively with one practice per market?**

5. **What kind of "done for you" and "done with you" services do you offer?**

6. **Do you offer or coordinate ongoing education or mastermind groups where I or a member of my practice can share ideas with other practices?**

7. **Do you offer a 100 percent money back results guarantee?**

**7 REASONS TO USE AN
OUTSIDE MARKETING EXPERT**

1. Your time is your inventory; you can only sell it once. Spend it on money-making activities if you can afford to pay someone to "make deposits" in your "future bank."
2. They create speed of implementation.
3. They help you fail fast and correct course.
4. Time is money. An expert's time, and fee, will be amortized over the life of the asset he creates for your practice.
5. They are unaffected by customary industry practices and therefore are unbiased; they view things objectively.
6. It allows you to extend your knowledge base to everyone they know.
7. Breakthroughs will typically always come from outside your industry.

8

BOOK RECAP,
i.e. 'CLIFF NOTES'

*"An organization's ability to learn,
and translate that learning into action rapidly,
is the ultimate competitive advantage."*
— Jack Welch

If you skipped through the rest of the book, then you've really missed the meat of the transformation we are trying to help you accomplish. But in case that's how you read, I'm including this very-abbreviated wrap-up along with a quick bit of advice — go back and read the book!

ABOUT ME

I have spent the last nine years of my life running my UPS Store franchises across the United States, something I never thought I would be doing because I went to school to study mechanical engineering and thought I would be designing cars for the rest of my life.

When I opened my first store, I was immediately successful, money was coming in, the balance sheet was strong, and within two years I had bought my second store. I thought I was the next Donald Trump.

Then, the bottom fell out. The economy slowed down and my first store—which was a little ATM— was forced to relocate because of upgrades to the site where it was located. At the time, I had no plan on how to turn things around. That was the first blow.

So I started spending more money "marketing" my stores because I saw we had declining customer counts. At that point, it doesn't matter how much your average sale is when customers do come to the store—if you don't have enough customers walking in, you will fall short of your sales goals.

Well, this went on for about two years and fortunately I did enough of the "right" things that we pulled through, and within one year of that I was in expansion mode again.

The following year, I opened or purchased another four stores. That is when all hell broke loose.

A double-dip recession in concert with new stores that were slowly starting to make money was more than I could financially bear. I had to do something ASAP because I didn't have enough money in the bank to make it through the next six months, much less the year.

That's when I found and started learning about marketing protocols. It was at that moment that I realized how little I really knew about marketing my stores and what a fool I had been, wasting tens of thousands of dollars on the wrong type of marketing for my small business.

Fortunately, after a very trying year and a few more missteps, I was able to stem the bleeding and begin on the road to recovery.

MAKING IT APPLICABLE

So what does this all have to do with you?

Well, if you picked up this book, it might be because you're going through what I went through a few years ago. If you're like I was at that point, you're looking for a lifeline, someone to help you and guide you. Your practice could also be doing great right now, but maybe your rate of growth has slowed down or even plateaued, maybe you have more competition now than you did five years ago and they're starting to impact your business. Maybe you're killing yourself working 12 to 14 hour days and seeing more patients than you're truly comfortable with because you're wearing a nice set of "golden handcuffs" that dictate how hard and long you have to work just to keep your current lifestyle and income level.

Whatever the reason, you're looking for something to reinvigorate your practice. Well you've come to the right place, your competitors aren't going to know what hit them. What do I know about a cosmetic practice? Admittedly, not very much.

What I do know a lot about is business and marketing a business.

I know that the heart of your practice is no different from any other business that exists in this world. You attract patients to your practice, you perform a service or deliver a product, and patients give you money in return.

The key component of that equation is the patients. Nothing happens until a patient walks in the door. You want to guarantee that patients not only walk in the door, but that the right kind of patients walk in the door. And you want to do this is the most reliable, repeatable, and profitable way possible, or else you'll slowly put yourself out of business.

You see, your business is an asset, quite possibly one of the biggest ones you'll ever own, maybe even bigger than your primary home. Failure to treat it as such and make decisions that will help the asset appreciate is a big mistake a lot of physicians make.

Have you ever asked yourself what do you I want to do with my practice once it's all said and done? Do you want to sell it? Do you want to pass it down? Do you want to close it? Do you want to use it as a source of continued income after you retire? Start with the end in mind and have a very clear picture of what you want that end to look like. If you want to do anything other than close it down, you need to be making decisions now and positioning your practice so that it grows in value.

MARKETING PROTOCOLS

Putting marketing protocols in place at your practice will help you grow its value.

The creation of reliable and repeatable protocols turn an expense — advertising — into an asset because you know what the return on investment (ROI) will be of everything you do. A predictable ROI will allow your practice to command a higher asking price come sale time or predictable income streams into retirement.

What's more having protocols in your practice will allow you to attract a better quality of patient that is not shopping based solely on fee. This allows you to have more work-life balance by spending less time at without worrying that revenue will decline. On the contrary you will be able to have more free time and make more money from seeing fewer patients.

A hidden benefit of these protocols is that they competition-proof your practice. Because your patient-generation protocols will become so complex and multi-stepped, you feasibly could lock all of your competitors in a room, show them exactly what you're doing and how you're doing it, and no one would copy you. They would say it's too hard or complex, they want to do what's easy.

The goal of your lead-generation protocols is to have suspect patients raise their hand indicating they're interested in your offer. You then bring them into a theoretical "room" and start to communicate with them and teach them about cosmetic procedures. You control what they see, read, and hear. Only you can let them in or out when you're ready to.

This whole process is done so that you can shift their buying criteria. Most of the time their primary method for comparing the practices is fee. They don't do this because they're penny pinchers, it's because they don't know any other way to compare them.

When you start educating them, you start to shift their buying criteria away from fee. You give them criteria that only your practice can meet 100 percent; this differentiates you and highlights your strengths versus all of your competitors.

Studies have shown that, at any given moment, for any given product or service, only 10 percent of the entire market is ready to buy now. Another 10 percent of that same market that will never buy, and a full 80 percent that have some level of interest in your product or service. Most practices fight tooth and nail for 10 percent and ignore the 80 percent. You are going to start focusing on creating protocols to capture a piece of that 80 percent in addition to a piece of the 10 percent.

If that 80 percent represented 1,000 patients, and you captured 20 percent, that's an additional 200 new patients. What would that do to your bottom line?

THE PROTOCOLS

What I'm proposing takes time, commitment, and dedication. It doesn't rely strictly on social media and online marketing. It's a mixture of media, some of which you're already familiar with, but might've discounted years ago.

You're going to take your online leads offline and your offline leads online. You're going to use direct mail, space advertising, Facebook, pay per click, and even billboards.

Currently, there is a huge gap between what consultants tell you should do and what actually works. Yes, online does work, but it doesn't beat offline direct mail. What's the first thing you do every morning when you wake up or maybe when you first walk into your practice? You check your email or you hop online and the bombardment begins. Online you push your way through pop-ups, paid search results, and annoying pre-video ads. At this point they have become white noise in the online world.

On the flip side what's the first thing you or your spouse or partner do when you get home? Check your mail, right? You interact with every piece of mail that comes in and make a decision of trashing it, opening it later, or opening it immediately.

You might say it's not very different to email or online right, but the truth is you physically inspected the mail piece, flipped it over, maybe even peeked inside. With the inbox getting more and more cluttered every day, and your mailbox getting emptier and emptier it's not hard to stand out offline

If you believe me that offline has huge potential, is untapped, and that you're going to let everyone else follow the pied piper "gurus" leading everyone off an online cliff, what else are you going to do?

A couple of tried-and-true-strategies have worked like a charm for me and my clients. One of the biggest mistakes all practices make is they have an obsessive focus on getting new patients. Obsessive is derived from the word obsession, which means an idea or thought that continually preoccupies or intrudes on a person's mind. The idea of new patients is so pervasive in their minds that they completely forget or abandon the existing customers they already have.

The easiest sale you will ever make is the repeat sale, period. Don't ignore your existing customers, they have already told you with their wallets that they like and trust you. If you believe wholeheartedly that the service you're providing will better their lives, then it is your responsibility to let them know.

I encourage all practices to run periodic lost or dormant patient reactivation campaigns. One such campaign that we run yearly returns at least $1.75 for every dollar we spend on it. It's our "secret-letter" campaign.

If you want to **get a copy of this lost customer campaign**, have your office manager **fax "lost customer sample" on practice letterhead to 1-888-316-5887** and I'll be happy to get it out to you. You can also **request a sample at my website, www.mgmca.com/lostcustomersample** and I'll send you one in the mail so you get the "full" lost-customer experience.

This campaign works for two reasons:
- It is personalized to the patient or prospect.
- It is different from anything else they'll get in their mailbox.

A second strategy that works well with both existing and unconverted patients is physical newsletters. As of this writing my stores were seeing a return of approximately almost $30 for every dollar spent on this old-fashioned marketing tool. Not bad for a tactic that many of today's online only gurus will tell you is dead and that nobody uses anymore.

> **To get a sample of the newsletter I use** that's bringing close to $30 for every $1 we spend on it, have your office manager **fax "newsletter sample" on practice letterhead to 1-888-316-5887** and I'll be happy to get my template out to you. You can also **request it at my website, www.mgmca.com/newslettersample**, and I'll send one via email.

Typically, newsletters wind up hanging around a person's home for a couple of months after they have been received and read.

The trick to a newsletter is that its content needs to be personal and not strictly clinical. Inject aspects of your own life and feature yourself, your family, and members of your practice heavily. This helps existing patients and prospects relate to you and see you as just another member of their community, not only as the awesome surgeon they previously knew you as.

You can have a small section in the newsletter where you talk about procedures or technologies, but do it in an educational way using language and examples that laymen can understand.

Also create a prospects only newsletter that you send to your patients that didn't schedule as an excuse to stay in contact with them for 12 months. Insider tip: Have two versions of these same newsletters with identical content, but with different tracking phone numbers for recipients to call to request more information so that you can measure ROI. The content of these prospects newsletters can be canned, so they can be reused year after year.

Finally, the strategy that will almost never be trumped by your competitors just because of its sheer difficulty is writing a book. I'm talking about a lead generation book to give to prospective patients that positions you as the local "author" and gives you instant authority and celebrity.

The goal of these efforts is to differentiate yourself by using the A.C.E.

formula, or authority, celebrity, and exclusivity.

When you're an authority on any topic, you by default become a celebrity. I'm not talking about celebrity like Tom Cruise or Oprah Winfrey. I'm talking about a celebrity no one outside of your market or niche might have heard of, but a celebrity that has huge name recognition to your market.

Once you've established your authority and celebrity, you can introduce exclusivity to your practice. As a result you can charge higher fees and still have a steady line of prospective patients eager to work with you at almost any price. This is when you have really taken your practice and repositioned it in such a way that your competitors will have a very difficult time trying to duplicate it.

The last tactic I highly recommend is the creation of a cosmetic surgery buying guide. When creating this buying guide you do so in such a way that your practice is the only one that can meet all the criteria. Typically, patients that are in the final stages of research will request and use the guide, and it allows patients to compare practices on something other than fees.

Before they have this guide, patients often base their decision solely on fee since they don't know how else to compare two seemingly identical practices.

YOU MAKE THE SALE

I also prospose that you, the physician, be the person to close all consultations and go over treatment plans. If you've done all the pre-work before a patient shows up at your practice, then closing a consultation should be no problem. It'll become selling without selling. Your authority, celebrity, and exclusivity should've already educated your prospect that your practice is not going to be the cheapest, but it is going to be the one best-suited to take care of her.

As part of this selling process, once the patient is in your office, you should go over these three key points: burning reason, future pace, objections.

First, have your patient verbalize to you their burning reason for wanting this procedure. Next, you need to future pace your patients and have them envision their life after their treatment is completed and they've undergone their transformation. Last, you need deal with objections, which are really just unanswered questions.

Whatever you do, do not haggle over fee. Instead, acknowledge the patient's concerns and suggest a more affordable alternative.

I also highly recommend that you have and make use of a "closing room" that is not your actual office or an examination room. The *only* use of this room is to close a consultation, *nothing* else. You would be surprised how many practices pay no attention to this *huge* detail and will attempt to close a consultation in an office with overflowing stacks of paper or in an impersonal exam room.

Remember that everything in your practice speaks. So have two or three strategically placed pieces on the wall of your closing room that a patient can examine when you excuse yourself for a minute. My suggestions would be any award you might've received, a picture of you and your family with a dog (if you don't have one, borrow one), and maybe a nice emotional testimonial letter with photo nicely framed.

Also at closing make sure you have nothing in between you and your patient. Pull up a chair and sit close to them as you go over treatment. You want your heart lines to be perfectly aligned. Selling is transference of emotion, so make sure nothing is in the way of you and your patient, not even your desk.

As your authority, celebrity, and exclusivity continue to grow throughout the community, you or your practice partners need to become the face of your practice. Initially this might feel awkward because essentially you may be exposing different aspects of your life to the public. But by allowing people into a portion of your personal life you will accomplish two things: one, you will allow them to see how a successful doctor lives and how interesting his work is; two, you will show people that you're just like everyone else in their community. This will make your practice more approachable without it reducing your exclusivity. We all want to do business with people we know, like, and trust, this allows people to do just that.

Eventually however you and everyone else in your partnership needs to take a step to the side and have the practice itself become the celebrity. You want the pieces inside of it to be almost interchangeable because the practice itself is a beacon for quality and excellence. This will also curb your dependence on any one specific person in the practice.

This strategy takes a little longer to develop, but it will help you break the work/money link you currently have with your practice—you know, the one that says you only make money when you're the one seeing all the patients. It will give you the independence and autonomy you've worked so hard to achieve.

The most important piece of all that has been discussed in this book is probably the most obvious, you have to implement concurrently, not sequentially. You need to carve out at least two to four hours every day for the first six months to work on your practice instead of just in it.

THE REVENUE EQUATION

In the beginning, implementing these marketing protocols may mean lost revenue if you work on them during the workday.

Let's say your time is worth at a minimum $250 per hour, and you're investing two hours every week for six months to get this going. That's equivalent to an approximate investment of $12,000. If your average cosmetic procedure is $3,000 on the low side, you would have to schedule just four additional procedures in one year to recuperate that investment. With even a bare bones marketing protocol in place, you should be able to do this easily.

Aside from that, you'll have a protocol that you can reuse for years.

If you simply don't have the time for do-it-yourself marketing, consider bringing in an outside consultant to help guide you through creating your first protocol and shorten the implementation curve.

Here's a short checklist to help you when interviewing prospective consultants.

> A printable, digital version of this can be found at
> **www.mgmca.com/guide**

These are the seven questions all marketing consultants must be able to answer.

1. Do you currently have marketing protocols in your business to generate new and repeat business? Tell me about it.

You need a consultant that understands that marketing is more than just a shotgun, feast-or-famine, slash-and-burn event. You need a partner who will help you generate a steady stream of new and repeat business. Someone who works to attract only the best customers for their business. Someone who works smarter not harder. Key words or phrases they might use if they have no marketing protocols in place are:

- Cold-call, network, or canvas
- Social media, Facebook, or Twitter
- I'm out on calls all day.
- What we do is different.
- We work with anyone.

2. Have you been trained by a pioneer and an authority in marketing and do you belong to his insider's circle?

What you're looking for here is someone who has learned from the best in the industry. By doing this you leapfrog years of trial and error with the wrong partner and use only strategies and tactics that have been proven to make money. You want a partner that's going to offer direct, unlimited access to the guru himself by belonging to their inner circle.

3. How are you continually expanding your knowledge? And how are you using what you have learned?

What you drill them on is how they are using what they're learning to help their clients make money as well. It's a partnership, remember? This takes a lot of out-of-the-box thinking.

A narrow, unimaginative mind always looks for the easiest answer—the path of least resistance. As I mentioned before, easy gives you no defense against competition. The harder something is to duplicate, the more built-in defenses it will have and the longer you will have the edge. Breakthroughs almost always come from outside, from borrowing and adapting.

Always look for a partner that is continually growing, not just to pad their own wallet, but to pad the wallets of their clients. Someone who is spreading the wealth.

4. Do you partner exclusively with one practice per market?

I won't beat around the bush here. It's unethical and a conflict of interest to have more than one horse in your stable. Anyone who argues the opposite is dead wrong.

Remember, this is a partnership. One where both parties get positive results out of it and are loyal to each other. If not, who gets the killer new marketing idea? You can't cut the baby in half.

You want a true partner, someone who is as committed to your success as you are. You want an extension of your practice that will be with you no matter how much you paid them last month. Someone who will be there as long as your relationship is as beneficial for you as it is for them. Then and only then can you really call it a partnership.

Warning: Anyone who starts any type of relationship with a long, undefined contract is probably only looking out for themselves. They are telling you from the very beginning that if things go bad they will collect! Doesn't exactly scream partnership does it?

5. What kind of "done for you" and "done with you" services do you offer?

The kind of "done for you" and "done with you" service I'm talking about is capturing all of your leads, prospects, and suspects. Delivering leads is easy. What do you do about the prospects and suspects that don't exactly scream out to you that they're interested?

Remember that at any given time only about 10 percent of your target market is ready to buy immediately. Another 10 percent is not and will never be interested. So what do you do about the other 80 percent that has some level of interest?

This is where the real money is made. Moving these 80 percent from suspects to prospects to leads then finally to patients is what a "done for you" and "done with you" service is all about.

The right partner understands these facts and will help you capture as much or as little of that remaining 80 percent as you want. Failure to follow up is failing to plan. Failure to plan is planning to fail.

6. Do you offer or coordinate ongoing education or mastermind groups where I or a member of my practice can share ideas with other practices?

A true partner should not be afraid to lift the veil and let you peak behind the curtain to show you how they do what they do. On the contrary, a true partner should help you make the connections you need to be more successful. Have I mentioned that almost all business breakthroughs come from outside their industry? There's real power in mastermind groups. Harness it.

7. Do you offer a 100 percent money back results guarantee?

Talk is cheap. A potential partner that is not willing to lay it all out on the line and back his claims is either:

- Not very good at what they do.
- Greedy and hates losing money, which is probably because they're not very good at what they do.
- Is not really interested in forming any sort of long-term partnership with you and your practice.

Now that you have your buying guide—and most importantly, now that you have a better understanding of the significance of marketing protocols for your practice—I would like to extend you a one-time offer as show of gratitude for purchasing and reading my book.

I invite you to learn more about how we can help your practice differentiate itself from the others, attract more of your ideal patients, and enjoy a better work-life balance without your practice's bottom-line suffering.

I am offering to work with you and **help you implement your first marketing protocol with no upfront fee.** I'm willing to put my money where my mouth is, and if you don't make any money, I don't make any money.

Why am I doing this? Well because I've found that the majority of physicians, and business owners for that matter, do little or nothing to implement what they've learned after reading a book, attending a seminar, or taking a class. They get a ton of notes and ideas then life happens when they return to their practice. They get busy, their staff talks them out of it, or they try to find a "better" time to implement. The excuses go on and on. I offer you speed of implementation, and money loves speed.

If you would like **to take me up on this offer please call fax "cosmetics book diagnostic consultation" on your practice letter head to 1-888-316-5887** to schedule a diagnostic call with me so I can learn a little bit more about your practice and your long term goals.

Please be sure to include an email address where we can contact you directly and a best time to call to schedule the appointment.

While scheduling the call we will take a $300 deposit that is 100 percent refundable after we've had the call.

Why the fee? Two reasons: One, my time is valuable and have limited inventory so I have to place a value on it regardless of what I do; and two, it guarantees that you will show up for the call—this goes back to my limited inventory, I can't resell that hour to someone if I've set it aside for you.

After scheduling the call you'll receive a short five-question survey so I can learn a little bit more about your practice and determine if you're a good candidate for my help. If we're a fit, then I'll be happy to get to work with you immediately.

If this still **sounds like too big of a commitment**, I understand. Remember: Only 10 percent are ready to take you up on any offer right now, that's why **I have something for you as well.**

You can **go to www.mgmca.com/toolkit and download our cosmetic practice makeover toolkit.** In it you will find samples and templates of all the different pieces and strategies I discussed in this book. Many of these are near fill-in-the-blank pieces where, with some minor modifications, you can start using them immediately. They are **100 percent copyright free.**

I only ask two things: that you don't use them exactly as you get them in order to set your practice apart from others who take me up on this offer; and that you **share your results with me by faxing them to 1-888-316-5887 or by emailing them to info@mgmca.com**. That way, I can either make them stronger or, with your permission, I can share your successes with other like-minded physicians that are just starting and need encouragement.

9

FINAL THOUGHTS

*"Being good in business is
the most fascinating kind of art.
Making money is art and working is art
and good business is the best art."*
— Andy Warhol

Now you're ready to go out and transform your practice. Although this book is by no means all-encompassing, what I have given you is the foundation upon which you can build great things if you dedicate a little time to it each day.

The key takeaway should be that if you want to get different outcomes from what you're currently getting, you need to stop doing what you're currently doing. If you haven't thought about what kind of end you want for your practice, now would be a great time to contemplate that, especially if you're at a crossroads in your career and can go in any direction you choose.

You also need to take a long, hard look at your own practice and, as noted author Napoleon Hill suggested, have "accurate thinking." You have to analyze all the facts and decide which will help you reach the end you had in mind. The ones that you can use are important and relevant; the ones you can't use should be thrown away and forgotten. This will not only help you simplify your mission but it will help give you clarity of thought and a filter through which all decisions must pass before you act on them.

What I have shared with you in this book is light years ahead of the way your competitors think. It's up to you to continue to develop these skills and truly differentiate yourself from all of them. Again, **if you found this book useless and a waste of your time and money, I invite you to call me directly at 1-915-241-7470 and request a full refund plus $100 just for your trouble**. I give you such a strong guarantee on the content of this book because I trust you to not take advantage of me and my offer and because I am that confident that it will help you.

It has been my mission ever since I pulled myself up from near failure a few years back to share my discoveries with other business owners and entrepreneurs to help them transform their business. The cosmetic surgery industry is one that deals in the ultimate transformation, that of the human body, and it is the primary reason why I am so drawn to it. You could say I help transform those who transform.

Whatever road you now decide to take you will have better tools in your toolbox. Good luck and Godspeed.

"Making excuses and making money is mutually exclusive."
–Dan Kennedy

About the Author

"Life is a series of missed opportunities,
so go for yours."
— *Victor Urbina*

Victor Urbina was born and raised in El Paso, Texas, and has lived there for the majority of his life. He has been an entrepreneur since childhood, starting his own soda stand in the heart of downtown El Paso at the age of 11 that he operated for three years. He attended The University of Texas at El Paso where he received a bachelor's degree in mechanical engineering.

He has worked for some of the biggest companies in their respective industries. He started his engineering career in the corporate world at Applied Materials in Silicon Valley and later changed industries by going to work for General Motors in Kansas City. While still at General Motors, he received a Master of Business Administration, also from The University of Texas at El Paso, working and studying concurrently. His tenure in corporate America helped him realize that he was an entrepreneur at heart and provoked him to return to his roots.

Victor opened his first UPS Store franchise in 2006 at Fort Bliss Military Base in El Paso, and within four months the store was turning a monthly profit. By late 2008, he purchased his second store, also in El Paso, and quickly turned a struggling store into a profitable one by restructuring operations and increasing customer sales. In 2011, he began a national expansion and opened three stores over a period of 15 months. Those stores are located in: Albuquerque, New Mexico; Fort Lee Military Base in Virginia; and Colonial

Heights, Virginia.

The lessons Victor has learned in business have come the hard way at times. Most notably, a few years ago, he was on the brink of losing all of his business. He quickly had to learn how to effectively market his businesses and so began what has now become a lifelong journey and one that brings him tremendous joy and challenge. Within sixteen months of undertaking this new challenge he was able to bring his businesses back onto better financial footing.

As result of his success he was asked by colleagues and other business owners to help them with their own business marketing. The lessons that he learned during his lean times are the ones he now shares with them.

Victor has always been fascinated with medicine and more specifically plastic surgery. It was because of this fascination that he realized that the cosmetic plastic surgery market was no different from his own retail background and that they could benefit from marketing their services more efficiently to have a better lifestyle and more autonomy.

Today, Victor and his wife, Georgialina, who holds a Ph.D. in immunology and is an associate research professor doing lymphoma research at The University of Texas at El Paso, live in El Paso, Texas along with their four dogs and four cats.

Victor is actively involved in the community where he serves on multiple boards including the Boys and Girls Club, Community En Acción, and the Hispanic Chamber of Commerce. He was a board member on the Marketing Advisory Council for The UPS Store where he helped direct the $25 million-plus annual marketing and advertising budget to optimize ROI for all UPS Store franchisees. He is also the founder of "Photo With Santa Palooza" a yearly Christmastime event that gives low-income families in the community an opportunity to take a photo with Santa in exchange for a canned good.

Victor is proud of his Hispanic heritage and Mexican roots, but above all else, Victor is proud to be an El Pasoan.

¡Vamos Raza!

Made in the USA
Lexington, KY
27 October 2016